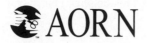 

PERIOPERATIVE NURSING CLINICS

Infection Control

George Allen, RN, PhD, CNOR, CIC
Guest Editor

Patricia C. Seifert, RN, MSN, CNOR, CRNFA, FAAN
Consulting Editor

June 2008 • Volume 3 • Number 2

SAUNDERS

An Imprint of Elsevier, Inc.
PHILADELPHIA   LONDON   TORONTO   MONTREAL   SYDNEY   TOKYO

W.B. SAUNDERS COMPANY
A Division of Elsevier Inc.

Elsevier Inc. • 1600 John F. Kennedy Boulevard • Suite 1800 • Philadelphia, Pennsylvania 19103-2899

http://www.periopnursing.theclinics.com

PERIOPERATIVE NURSING CLINICS
June 2008
Editor: Alexandra Gavenda

Volume 3, Number 2
ISSN 1556-7931
ISBN-13: 978-1-4160-5779-6
ISBN-10: 1-4160-5779-X

Perioperative Nursing Clinics (ISSN 1556-7931) is published quarterly by Elsevier, 360 Park Avenue South, New York, NY 10010. Months of issue are March, June, September and December. Business and Editorial Office: 1600 John F. Kennedy Blvd., Ste. 1800, Philadelphia, PA 19103-2899. Accounting and Circulation Offices: 6277 Sea Harbor Dr, Orlando, FL 32887-4800. Periodicals postage paid at New York, NY and at additional mailing offices.

POSTMASTER: Send change of address to *Perioperative Nursing Clinics*, Elsevier, Periodicals Department, 6277 Sea Harbor Dr, Orlando, FL 32887-4800. **Customer Service: 1-800-654-2452 (US). From outside the United States, call 1-407-563-6020. Fax: 1-407-363-9661. E-mail: JournalsCustomer Service-usa@elsevier.com.**

Printed in the United States of America.

CONSULTING EDITOR

PATRICIA C. SEIFERT, RN, MSN, CNOR, CRNFA, FAAN, Education Coordinator, Cardiovascular Operating Room, Inova Heart and Vascular Institute, Falls Church, Virginia

GUEST EDITOR

GEORGE ALLEN, RN, PhD, CNOR, CIC, Director of Infection Control, Downstate Medical Center, Brooklyn, New York

CONTRIBUTORS

AUDREY B. ADAMS, RN, BSN, MPH, CIC, Administrative Nurse Manage, Infection Control, Montefiore Medical Center, Bronx, New York

GEORGE ALLEN, RN, PhD, CNOR, CIC, Director of Infection Control, Downstate Medical Center, Brooklyn, New York

KEVIN CALDWELL, RN, BSN, CNOR, Clinical Instructor, Consortium of Workers Education, New York, New York

JANET P. HAAS, RN, DNSc, Associate Director, Infection Prevention and Control Department, New York University Medical Center, New York, New York

SANDRA HARDY, RN, MA, Infection Prevention and Control Department, New York University Medical Center, New York, New York

LUCILLE H. HERRING, RN, MS, CIC, Infection Control Nurse, Weiler Division, Montefiore Medical Center, Bronx, New York

MARY ANN MAGERL, RN, MA, CIC, Nurse Epidemiologist, Infection Control Department, Westchester Medical Center, Valhalla, New York

KATHI MULLANEY, BSN, MPH, CIC, Our Lady of Mercy Medical Center, Bronx, New York

CYNTHIA SPRY, RN, MA, MSN, CNOR, New York, New York

TANIA N. WILLIAMS, RN, MSN, Infection Prevention and Control Practitioner, Infection Prevention and Control Department, New York University Medical Center, New York, New York

CONTENTS

Hand Hygiene: A Patient Safety Issue in the Perioperative Environment 101
George Allen

Hand hygiene represents the single most important procedure in the health care milieu for preventing the transmission of infection. Although the perioperative environment is viewed as an area where all members of the surgical team religiously comply with the concept of surgical asepsis, compliance by all personnel may not be so rigorous for general day-to-day hand hygiene between each patient contact and contact with the environment. Providing the infrastructure and facilities, conducting observations, and posting compliance rates by disciplines in the perioperative setting are critical components in efforts to increase compliance with hand hygiene and consequently improve patient safety.

Is Hair Removal Necessary Before the Surgical Incision? 107
Audrey B. Adams

Two preoperative male patients are scheduled for elective coronary artery bypass procedures. Both patients have hairy chest. Surgeon A orders preoperative removal of hair for his patient directly before surgery with clippers, and surgeon B does not order hair removal for his patient. Based on the literature, which preoperative hair removal practice will be most beneficial to avoid a surgical site infection?

Preparing for the Patient Who Has Prion Disease 115
Cynthia Spry

The mention of Creutzfeldt-Jakob (CJD) disease can be cause for apprehension in those responsible for the patients and/or for those responsible for cleaning, disinfecting, or sterilizing devices, including surgical instruments, used on a known or suspected patient with this disease. Although CJD has been discussed in the medical literature for many years, it is only in the last 10 or so years that it has become a "hot topic."

FORTHCOMING ISSUES

RECENT ISSUES

ELSEVIER
SAUNDERS

Perioperative Nursing Clinics 3 (2008) ix–x

PERIOPERATIVE
NURSING
CLINICS

Foreword

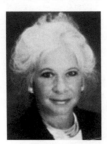

Patricia C. Seifert, RN, MSN, CNOR, CRNFA, FAAN
Consulting Editor

One technological advance— the introduction of the steam sterilizer in the 1880's [1]—ushered in the era of aseptic surgery. Infection had been one of the great barriers (in addition to pain, hemorrhage, and pneumothorax) to performing surgery effectively. With the introduction of sterilization, surgeons were able to achieve reproducible and successful outcomes more consistently, which not only significantly improved operative results, but also enhanced the stature of surgeons.

What is appreciated insufficiently is that the introduction of the steam sterilizer also put the nurse "on the map." Before the advent of sterilization (and greater control of potentially deadly environmental pathogens), the nurse's role was depicted largely as the application of cool cloths and warm hands. This does not denigrate the role of caring behaviors, rather, it stresses that nurses could be *proactive* as well as reactive in their care of patients.

The contemporary role of the nurse as a proactive "knowledge worker" is evident in the collection of articles on the subject of infection control. Guest Editor Dr. George Allen illustrates the broad array of interventions that have enabled nurses to protect their patients (and colleagues) from environmental pathogens, prevent transmission of communicable diseases, and develop safe practices to minimize the risk of infection. These are active, not passive, behaviors, and they attest to the leadership role of nurses within the current health care arena.

The articles in this issue address topics as basic as hand washing and hair removal; other topics, such as prion diseases and multi-drug resistant pathogens, are more complex. It is evident that if we are to serve as patient advocates, our knowledge of infection control must be broad and deep. Even subjects as mundane as sterilization, disinfection, sanitation, and facility construction require new and innovative ways to address the issues of safety and efficacy. Infection is associated with morbidity and mortality and also places considerable financial burden on health care institutions and patients.

Knowledge of infection control issues and the implementation of effective practices reflect a cornerstone of professional nursing. Dr. Allen and his coauthors have provided additional building blocks for perioperative nurses to highlight their knowledge and skill in the care of patients.

This will be my last *Foreword* as Consulting Editor of the *Perioperative Nursing Clinics*. It has been a privilege and a pleasure to serve as your editor and to provide issues of the *Perioperative Nursing Clinics* that have focused on multiple facets of key issues affecting perioperative nursing and health care in general. My vision as the first consulting editor was to select topics of

1556-7931/08/$ - see front matter © 2008 Elsevier Inc. All rights reserved.
doi:10.1016/j.cpen.2008.02.006

importance to readers and to highlight clinical, financial, professional, and other pertinent aspects of each subject. Our Guest Editors have provided excellent resources on the subjects of bariatric, vascular, and gynecologic surgery; evidence-based practice; the perioperative nursing data set; the future environment; advanced practice; electrosurgery; and in this issue—infection control. Great credit is due to the Guest Editors, experts in their field, who consistently gathered a team of authors who shared practical and intellectually sound information on their selected subject. I thank them.

Today's operative and invasive procedures are collaborative efforts designed to enhance patient care; the *Perioperative Nursing Clinics* reflects the expertise of many individuals and professional roles. It is my belief that perioperative nurses can only benefit from exposure to the ideas and knowledge of any individual who can contribute to a surgical patient's optimal outcome.

I thank my Elsevier counterparts: Maria Lorusso, who worked with me to create the first two issues of the Clinics, and Alexandra (Ali) Gavenda, who has provided invaluable assistance to develop and nurture all subsequent issues.

Patricia C. Seifert, RN, MSN, CNOR,
CRNFA, FAAN
Education Coordinator
Cardiovascular Operating Room
Inova Heart and Vascular Institute
3300 Gallows Road
Falls Church, VA 22042, USA

E-mail address: patricia.seifert@inova.com

Reference

[1] Alexander EL. Operating room technique. St. Louis: The C.V. Mosby Company; 1943. p. 35.

**ELSEVIER
SAUNDERS**

Perioperative Nursing Clinics 3 (2008) xi–xii

**PERIOPERATIVE
NURSING
CLINICS**

Preface

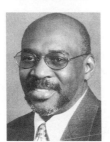

George Allen, RN, PhD, CNOR, CIC
Guest Editor

Health care associated infections (HAIs) are recognized now as a significant public health problem in the United States. It is estimated that approximately 2 million HAIs occur each year in the United States, accounting for an estimated 90,000 deaths and adding $4.5 to $5.7 billion in health care costs [1]. Approximately 38% of infections that occur in surgical patients are surgical site infections (SSIs), and 4% to 16% of all HAIs among all hospitalized patients are SSIs, and 2% to 5% of patients who have surgery will develop a SSI [2]. Additionally, personnel are at risk for occupational exposure to blood borne infections, including hepatitis B, hepatitis C, HIV [3], and other communicable diseases, including *Staphylococcus aureus* infections, tuberculosis, pertussis, measles, influenza, and varicella [4]. Consequently, in the health care milieu, infection control is accepted universally as an essential patient and personnel safety process requiring attention and compliance from all personnel. Therefore, the principal concern is ensuring safety by preventing the transmission of infections to patients and personnel.

In the perioperative environment there are numerous opportunities for infection control procedures to have a positive impact. The articles in this issue were selected not only to outline the critical importance of infection prevention and control activities in the perioperative environment, but also to highlight some basic infection prevention techniques for preventing infection in patients and personnel.

Personnel in the perioperative setting already are attuned to the importance of asepsis and sterility as vital infection control steps in preventing the spread of infections especially in patients whose intact skin has been intentionally breached by a surgical incision. The articles on hand hygiene review basic infection control principles for preventing infections in patients undergoing surgery. Articles included in this section are: my article, "A Patient Safety Issue for the Perioperative Setting;" Mullaney's article, "Sterilization and Disinfection in the Operating Room;" and Magerl's article, "Sanitation: Routine Cleaning Versus Terminal Cleaning."

doi:10.1016/j.cpen.2008.02.007

Additionally, Spry presents important information on protecting personnel when handling instruments after surgery has been conducted on patients who have a suspected prion disease. Allen and Caldwell describe rational procedures for safely caring for a patient who has infectious tuberculosis, and Adams eloquently reviews the issues of preoperative preparation of the patient, including a discussion on hair removal versus no hair removal. Herring outlines the importance of policies and procedures related to preventing transmission of hepatitis B infection, including hepatitis B vaccination, engineering controls, and work practice controls. Hardy and Haas discuss a proactive approach during construction and renovation activities to prevent invasive aspergillus infection among patients, and Williams and Haas review procedures for implementing contact isolation in the perioperative setting as multi-drug-resistant pathogens, including MRSA, become more prevalent.

In essence, these articles provide perioperative personnel with a telescopic view on the essential nature of infection control activities in the realm of facilitating and fostering the safety of patients and personnel throughout the perioperative experience.

George Allen, RN, PhD, CNOR, CIC
Director of Infection Control
Downstate Medical Center
450 Clarkson Avenue, Box 1187
Brooklyn, NY 11203-2056, USA

E-mail address: george.allen@downstate.edu

References

[1] Starfield B. Is US health really the best in the world? JAMA 2000;248:483–5.
[2] Mangram AJ, Horan TC, Pearson ML, et al. Guideline for prevention of surgical site infection, 1999. Hospital Infection Control Practices Advisory Committee. Infect Control Hosp Epidemiol 1999;20(4):247–78.
[3] Centers for Disease Control. Updated U.S. Public Health Service Guidelines for the management of occupational exposures to HBV, HCV, and HIV and recommendations for postexposure prophylaxis. MMWR 2001;50(RR-11).
[4] Boylard EA, Tablan OC, Williams WW, et al. Guideline for infection control in health care personnel, 1998. Am J Infect Control 1998;26:289–354.

Perioperative Nursing Clinics 3 (2008) 101–106

Hand Hygiene: A Patient Safety Issue in the Perioperative Environment

George Allen, RN, PhD, CNOR, CIC

Downstate Medical Center, 450 Clarkson Avenue, Box 1187, Brooklyn, NY 11203-2056, USA

Surgical asepsis in the perioperative environment is a concept that is universally understood and practiced by the surgical team before the incision is made. Components are the surgical scrub, adequate skin preparation of the patient, and the creation and maintenance of a sterile field. However, an equally important procedure before and after every patient contact throughout the health care milieu is hand hygiene. Like surgical asepsis in the perioperative environment, hand hygiene is a critical component for preventing the transmission of infection. Indeed, hand washing is the most important tool in controlling health care–associated infections [1] and the most important way to prevent the transmission of infection [2]. Health care personnel for more than a century have been taught that hands must be washed before and after each patient contact, when there is visible soiling, before donning gloves, and after removing gloves.

However estimates of compliance with hand hygiene in health care settings have not been heartening with rates below 60 percent. One study among staff in an intensive care unit (ICU) found an overall compliance rate of 72% after an educational program. The compliance rate was highest among nurses (97.5%), lowest among physicians (37.6%), and 47.7% among technicians [3]. Another study found baseline hand washing compliance before and after defined events was 9% and 22% respectively for health care workers in the medical ICU and 3% and 13% respectively in the cardiac surgery ICU [4]. Additionally, Larson and colleagues [5] found an overall compliance rate of 38.4% in pediatrics, and Pittet and colleagues [6] found an average adherence of 57% among physicians.

Glove use and hand washing

Current guidelines from the Occupational Safety and Health Administration (OSHA) Bloodborne Exposure Standard require the use of gloves when personnel are likely to have contact with blood, other potentially infectious material, mucous membranes, tissue, nonintact skin, when handling contaminated items or surfaces, and when performing vascular procedures, such as phlebotomies or insertions of intravascular catheters [7]. Gloves are an important barrier that can reduce hand contamination by approximately 80%. However, they break easily and can facilitate the proliferation of bacteria because the wearing of gloves creates a moist, warm environment for bacteria to rapidly grow and multiply [8]. Due to the large number of circulating bacteria that rapidly develops after donning gloves and the potential for the gloves to break, the likelihood of transmission and development of infection is increased. Gloves must never be used as a substitute for hand hygiene, because the risk is too great that a glove puncture or tear will occur, releasing bacteria that has multiplied inside the glove. Bacteria grow and multiply by binary fission every 6 minutes. Additionally, hand hygiene must also be performed when gloves are removed because the hands are now teeming with bacteria. Along with the need to routinely perform hand hygiene is the need to address issues related to the fingernails. Long and artificial fingernails have been implicated in the transmission of infection to patients and linked to death in the neonatal population. Additionally,

E-mail address: george.allen@downstate.edu

doi:10.1016/j.cpen.2008.01.003

the subungual areas of the hands are known to harbor bacteria in high concentrations, including coagulase-negative Staphylococci; gram-negative rods, including *Pseudomonas* sp; corynebacteria, and yeast. Thus, it is recommended that artificial nails not be used and that natural nails be kept to no more than one quarter inch in length [9]. Consequently, all institutions should have policies to ensure that personnel who have physical contact with patients wear no artificial nails and keep their nails neat and short, in addition to performing hand hygiene before and after each patient contact.

Hand hygiene methods

The classical method when performing hand hygiene involves using soap and water. Personnel are instructed to:

1. Turn the faucet on and adjust the temperature of the water to warm.
2. Wet hands.
3. Apply soap.
4. Vigorously rub all surfaces of the hands and fingers, between the web spaces, and under the nails for 15 seconds.
5. Rinse with water.
6. Dry thoroughly with a disposable towel, and use the towel to turn off the faucet.

The current hand hygiene recommendations from the Centers for Disease Control and Prevention aimed at improving adherence to hand hygiene now also recommend the use of waterless, alcohol-based hand hygiene products, which should be placed in convenient locations in patient care areas [2]. Alcohol-based waterless products are effective and can be used as long as hands are not visibly soiled, and as long as spore-forming organisms, such as *Clostridium difficile*, are not suspected. Because alcohol can support combustion, these hand hygiene products should not be placed over or next to sources of ignition, including electrical switches and outlets, lasers, or electrosurgical equipment [10]. The alcohol-based product must be applied thoroughly and uniformly, worked into the hands, and allowed to dry. Approximately 0.5 mL to 0.7 mL of most products is adequate for sanitizing the hands of most health care workers. Occasionally more of the product is needed to cover the entire hands.

The World Health Organization recognizes five sequential elements required for health care–associated pathogens, including multidrug resistant pathogens, such as methicillin-resistant *Staphylococcus aureus* and vancomycin-resistant enteroccus, to be transmitted from one patient to another on the hands of health care workers. They include:

1. The microorganisms are present on the skin of the patient, or have been shed onto inanimate objects in the patient's immediate environment.
2. The microorganisms must be transferred to the health care worker's hands.
3. The microorganisms must be capable of surviving for at least several minutes on the hands of the health care worker.
4. Hand washing and hand hygiene by the health care worker must be inadequate or not performed, or the agent for hand hygiene is inappropriate.
5. The contaminated hand or hands of the health care worker must come into direct contact with another patient or with an inanimate object that will come into direct contact with the patient [11].

This sequence of events is possible in any health care setting, including the perioperative environment for all members of the surgical team who may have contact with the patient. This means everyone from the unlicensed assistive personnel who transport the patient and assist with the transfer from the stretcher to the operating room table, to the holding area nurse who physically assesses the patient or inserts the peripheral intravenous catheter, or the anesthesia resident who assesses the oral cavity to determine the presence of dentures and loose teeth and the surgeon who marks the operative site before the patient enters the operating room. Additionally, when the patient is transported into the room where the surgical procedure will be done, there are further opportunities for unsterile personnel to have contact with the patient. Such contact requires hand hygiene. Examples of such contact include intubation of the patient by the anesthesia care provider and the handling of specimens and counting of used sponges by the circulating nurse.

Sinks are not always available in the perioperative areas where patient care activities require hand hygiene, such as inside the operating room or the holding area. Consequently, perioperative managers and administrators are making the alcohol-based waterless hand hygiene products available on the walls and in the corridors in these areas to ensure that adequate facilities are readily accessible to all personnel when hand hygiene is indicated. Appendix 1 provides a fact sheet on hand hygiene that can be posted as an educational tool for the perioperative team.

Indications for hand hygiene in the perioperative setting

In addition to the obvious instances when hand hygiene is necessary, such as checking for dentures and loose tooth, removing dentures, before conducting a physical examination on one patient, and before moving to another patient, hand hygiene is indicated in the perioperative setting in the following situations:

Before and after marking the incision site in the holding area
Before and after inserting intravenous lines in the holding area or in the operating room
Before intubating the patient, inserting the endotracheal tube, and especially at the end of the procedure after the gloves are removed
Before and after inserting urinary catheters and after removing bedpans and urinals
After contact with nonintact skin, tissue, and mucous membranes
After counting used sponges
After handling specimens
After removing dressings
After removing gloves and other personal protective equipment

Compliance with hand hygiene protocol is a critical step in preventing the transmission of infections. Indeed, according to the Joint Commission, it is a patient safety issue falling under their National Patient Safety Goals [12]. Health care institutions, to maintain Joint Commission accreditation, engender patient safety, and prevent transmission of infection, must therefore enforce compliance with hand hygiene requirements. Consequently, monitoring hand hygiene is an essential step in any hand hygiene program.

Monitoring hand hygiene

Health care institutions must develop institution-wide programs for assessing compliance with hand hygiene and implement procedures for improvement when indicated. Activities to ensure compliance with hand hygiene procedures might include:

Monitoring and recording adherence to hand hygiene by ward, service, or personnel type
Providing feedback to health care workers about their performance
Monitoring the volume of soap and alcohol-based products used
Monitoring adherence to policies on wearing artificial nails

Indeed, most institutions have programs that monitor personnel and document and report back to their employees their hand hygiene compliance rates by service, unit, and discipline. However, such programs are not common in the perioperative environment. Perioperative managers have a primary responsibility to patients and personnel to ensure that procedures are in place, such as procedures related to compliance with hand hygiene protocols, to reduce the potential for the transmission of infections [13]. Consequently, they should routinely assess the hand hygiene compliance rate of the surgical team, nurses, surgeon, technicians, and other unlicensed assistive personnel; inform personnel about those rates; and develop and implement corrective actions when the rates are poor. Appendix 2 provides an example of a monitoring tool that can be easily adapted to any perioperative setting to collect the data needed to determine the hand hygiene compliance rate by categories of personnel.

Assuring patient safety through hand hygiene

The development of health care–associated infections (HAI) is a patient safety issue. The Centers for Disease Control and Prevention estimates that 2 million patients in the United States develop an HAI each year, and more than 90,000 to 100,000 die as a result [14]. The key to preventing transmission of infections in the health care system, including the perioperative setting, is compliance with hand hygiene. It is imperative that all levels of health care workers who may have physical contact with the patient receive education on hand hygiene so that they understand that hand hygiene is the most important procedure for preventing the spread of infections. Additionally, facilities for hand hygiene should be readily accessible to all personnel. In the perioperative environment, where hand washing sinks are not appropriate in certain locations, then the alcohol-based waterless product must be made available. These can be mounted on walls in rooms where surgical procedures are performed, in the holding areas, and in corridors. Additionally, the compliance rate of personnel must be monitored and information must be posted and made available to the staff. Disciplines found to have low compliance rates must be reeducated.

Appendix 1

Hand hygiene guidelines fact sheet

- Improved adherence to hand hygiene (ie, hand washing or use of alcohol-based hand rubs) has been shown to terminate outbreaks of infection in health care facilities, to reduce transmission of antimicrobial resistant organisms (eg, methicillin resistant staphylococcus aureus), and reduce overall infection rates.
- The Centers for Disease Control and Prevention is releasing guidelines to improve adherence to hand hygiene in health care settings. In addition to traditional hand washing with soap and water, the Centers for Disease Control and Prevention is recommending the use of alcohol-based hand rubs by health care personnel for patient care because they address some of the obstacles that health care professionals face when taking care of patients.
- Hand washing with soap and water remains a sensible strategy for hand hygiene in non–health care settings and is recommended by the Centers for Disease Control and Prevention and other experts.
- When health care personnel's hands are visibly soiled, they should wash with soap and water.
- The use of gloves does not eliminate the need for hand hygiene. Likewise, the use of hand hygiene does not eliminate the need for gloves. Gloves reduce hand contamination by 70% to 80%, prevent cross-contamination, and protect patients and health care personnel from infection. Hand rubs should be used before and after each patient just as gloves should be changed before and after contact with each patient.
- When using an alcohol-based hand rub, apply product to palm of one hand and rub hands together, covering all surfaces of hands and fingers, until hands are dry. Note that the volume needed to reduce the number of bacteria on hands varies by product.
- Alcohol-based hand rubs significantly reduce the number of microorganisms on skin, are fast acting, and cause less skin irritation than soap and water.
- Health care personnel should avoid wearing artificial nails and keep natural nails less than one quarter of an inch long if they care for patients at high risk of acquiring infections (eg, patients in intensive care units or in transplant units).
- When evaluating hand hygiene products for potential use in health care facilities, administrators or product selection committees should consider the relative efficacy of antiseptic agents against various pathogens and the acceptability of hand hygiene products by personnel. Characteristics of a product that can affect acceptance and therefore usage include its smell, consistency, color, and the effect of dryness on hands.
- As part of these recommendations, the Centers for Disease Control and Prevention is asking health care facilities to develop and implement a system for measuring improvements in adherence to these hand hygiene recommendations. Some suggested activities for monitoring, measuring, enforcing, and encouraging adherence to hand hygiene recommendations include periodic monitoring of hand hygiene adherence and providing feedback to personnel regarding their performance, monitoring the volume of alcohol-based hand rub used per 1000 patient days, monitoring adherence to policies dealing with wearing artificial nails, and performing focused assessments of the adequacy of health care personnel hand hygiene when outbreaks of infection occur.
- Allergic contact dermatitis due to alcohol hand rubs is very uncommon. However, with increasing use of such products by health care personnel, it is likely that true allergic reactions to such products will occasionally be encountered.
- Alcohol-based hand rubs take less time to use than traditional hand washing. In an 8-hour shift, an intensive care unit nurse will save about 1 hour by using an alcohol-based hand rub.
- These guidelines should not be construed to legalize product claims that are not allowed by a Food and Drug Administration product approval by the Food and Drug Administration's Over-the-Counter Drug Review. The recommendations are not intended to apply to consumer use of the products discussed.

Adapted from Centers for Disease Control and Prevention. Hand hygiene guidelines fact sheet. Available at: http://www.cdc.gov/od/oc/media/pressrel/fs021025.htm. Accessed February 19, 2008; with permission.

Appendix 2
Perioperative hand hygiene monitoring form

PERIOPERATIVE HAND HYGIENE MONITORING FORM

AREA/ROOM---------------- TIME---------------- MONTH/YEAR ---------------- SURVEYOR ----------------

#	TYPE OF HEALTH CARE WORKER						HAND HYGIENE BEFORE CONTACT			HAND HYGIENE AFTER CONTACT			COMMENTS
	Surgeon	Anesthesia	Nurse	SurgTech	UAP	Other	ALC	Soap	N	ALC	Soap	N	
1	Surgeon	Anesthesia	Nurse	SurgTech	UAP	Other	ALC	Soap	N	ALC	Soap	N	
2	Surgeon	Anesthesia	Nurse	SurgTech	UAP	Other	ALC	Soap	N	ALC	Soap	N	
3	Surgeon	Anesthesia	Nurse	SurgTech	UAP	Other	ALC	Soap	N	ALC	Soap	N	
4	Surgeon	Anesthesia	Nurse	SurgTech	UAP	Other	ALC	Soap	N	ALC	Soap	N	
5	Surgeon	Anesthesia	Nurse	SurgTech	UAP	Other	ALC	Soap	N	ALC	Soap	N	
6	Surgeon	Anesthesia	Nurse	SurgTech	UAP	Other	ALC	Soap	N	ALC	Soap	N	
7	Surgeon	Anesthesia	Nurse	SurgTech	UAP	Other	ALC	Soap	N	ALC	Soap	N	
8	Surgeon	Anesthesia	Nurse	SurgTech	UAP	Other	ALC	Soap	N	ALC	Soap	N	
9	Surgeon	Anesthesia	Nurse	SurgTech	UAP	Other	ALC	Soap	N	ALC	Soap	N	
10	Surgeon	Anesthesia	Nurse	SurgTech	UAP	Other	ALC	Soap	N	ALC	Soap	N	
11	Surgeon	Anesthesia	Nurse	SurgTech	UAP	Other	ALC	Soap	N	ALC	Soap	N	
12	Surgeon	Anesthesia	Nurse	SurgTech	UAP	Other	ALC	Soap	N	ALC	Soap	N	
13	Surgeon	Anesthesia	Nurse	SurgTech	UAP	Other	ALC	Soap	N	ALC	Soap	N	
14	Surgeon	Anesthesia	Nurse	SurgTech	UAP	Other	ALC	Soap	N	ALC	Soap	N	
15	Surgeon	Anesthesia	Nurse	SurgTech	UAP	Other	ALC	Soap	N	ALC	Soap	N	
	TOTAL ENCOUNTERS/OBSERVATIONS: Surgeon Anesthesia Nurse SurgTech Other TOTAL						TOTAL #						%ADHERENCE/COMPLIANCE: Total # YES ÷ Total # of ENCOUNTERS X 100

Surgeon = attending, fellow, resident, PA, med stud; Anesthesia = attending, resident, CRNA, **N** = RN, LPN, RNFA, UAP = Un-licensed assistive personnel; Other = environmental services, transporter

Hand hygiene before/after: ALC = alcohol-based hand rub; Soap = hand washing with soap and water for 15 seconds

References

[1] Nystrom B. Impact of handwashing on mortality in intensive care: examination of the evidence. Infect Control Hosp Epidemiol 1994;15:435–6.

[2] Boyce JM, Pittet D. Guidelines for hand hygiene in health-care settings: recommendations of the Healthcare Infection Control Advisory Committee and the HIPAC/SHEA/APIC/ISDA Hand Hygiene Task Force. MMWR Morb Mortal Wkly Rep 2005; 51:1–45.

[3] Panhotra BR, Saxena AK, Al-Ghandi AM. The effect of a continuous educational program on hand-washing compliance among healthcare workers in an intensive care unit. British Journal of Infection Control 2004;5(3):15–8.

[4] Bischott WE, Reynolds TM, Sessler CN, et al. Handwashing compliance by healthcare workers: the impact of introducing an accessible alcohol based antiseptic. Arch Intern Med 2000;160: 1017–21.

[5] Larson EL, Albrecht S, O'Keefe M. Hand hygiene behavior in a pediatric emergency department and a pediatric intensive care unit: comparison of use of two dispenser systems. Am J Crit Care 2005;14: 304–11.

[6] Pittet D, Simon A, Hugonnet S, et al. Hand hygiene among physicians: performance, belief, and perceptions. Ann Intern Med 2004;141(1):1–8.

[7] Occupational Safety and Health Administration (OSHA). Occupational exposure to bloodborne pathogens; final rule. Fed Regist 1991;66:64004–182.

[8] Hand hygiene guidelines fact sheet. Centers for Disease Control and Prevention, Office of Communication. Available at: http://www.cdc.gov/od/oc/media/pressrel/fs021025.htm. Accessed January 27, 2008.

[9] Boyce JM, Pittet D. Guideline for hand hygiene in health-care settings. Recommendations of the Healthcare Infection Control Practices Advisory Committee and HICPAC/SHEA/APIC/IDSA Hand Hygiene Task Force. MMWR 2002;51:1–45.

[10] AORN guidance statement: fire prevention in the operating room. In: Standards and recommended practices and guidelines. Denver (CO): AORN, Inc; 2005. p. 143–51.

[11] World Health Organization, WHO guideline on hand hygiene in health care (advanced draft). 2005;10: 10–1. Available at: http://www.who.int/patientsafety/events/05/HH_en.pdf.

[12] Joint Commission. National patient safety goals. Available at: http://www.jointcommission.org/PatientSafety/NationalPatientSafetyGoals/08_hap_npsgs.htm.

[13] Allen G. Hand hygiene, an essential process in the OR. AORN J Guest Editorial 2005;82(4):561–2.

[14] Connolly C. Data show scourge of hospital infection. Washington Post 2005. Available at: http://www.washingtonpost.com/wp-dyn/content/article/2005/07/12/AR2005071201555.html.

**ELSEVIER
SAUNDERS**

Perioperative Nursing Clinics 3 (2008) 107–113

PERIOPERATIVE
NURSING
CLINICS

Is Hair Removal Necessary Before the Surgical Incision?

Audrey B. Adams, RN, BSN, MPH, CIC

Infection Control, Montefiore Medical Center, 111 E. 210th Street, Bronx, NY 10467, USA

Two preoperative male patients are scheduled for elective coronary artery bypass procedures. Both patients have hairy chest. Surgeon A orders preoperative removal of hair for his patient directly before surgery with clippers, and surgeon B does not order hair removal for his patient. Based on the literature, which preoperative hair removal practice will be most beneficial to avoid a surgical site infection (SSI)?

In this era of patient safety and prevention of surgical site infections, the issue of preoperative hair removal is discussed. Removal of hair before surgery has been the subject of numerous studies, starting in 1971 [1] and continuing through 2002, 2005, and 2007 with systematic literature reviews [2–4]. These studies are the source of current recommendations and regulatory mandates. The 1999 Centers for Disease Control (CDC) Guideline for Prevention of Surgical Site Infection [5] has two recommendations for preoperative hair removal: (1) it should not be performed unless the hair at or around the incision site would interfere with the operation, (2) if hair is removed, it should be performed immediately before the operation, preferably with electric clippers. Both of these are CDC Category 1A recommendations strongly recommended for implementation and supported by well-designed experimental, clinical, or epidemiologic studies.

Although the above recommendations have become the standard of practice, there remains controversy on the quality, study design, and findings of many studies on preoperative hair removal. Findings of three systematic reviews will be presented, along with a discussion of preoperative hair removal involving neurosurgical patients and the results of a small survey of hair

E-mail address: aadams@montefiore.org

removal practice by attending surgeons at a large voluntary teaching hospital in New York City.

Systematic literature reviews

The first systematic literature review published in 2002 was conducted in part as an effort to answer the question, to what extent was the CDC guideline for preoperative hair removal based on a systematic search of all relevant literature and a subsequent critical literature appraisal [2]. The authors stated that the CDC guideline did not describe the methods and search strategies of literature to generate the guideline. Therefore, before adopting the CDC guideline, the Norwegian Centre for Health Technology Assessment decided to systematically search and appraise relevant literature to compare their conclusions with those of the CDC. Seven electronic databases were used to search for scientific articles that dealt with preoperative hair removal and SSIs.

There were 120 articles identified that dealt with preoperative hair removal and SSIs. CDC articles cited in their guideline that were not found in the searches were included and assessed. The article searches ended in December 1999. The studies were divided into the following six groups: shaving compared with no hair removal; shaving compared with clipping; shaving compared with depilation; timing of preoperative hair removal with razor or clippers; and wet and dry shaving. Each of the studies was also categorized into various levels by type of documentation (Recommendations from the US Agency for Healthcare Policy and Research).

The authors found that studies that compared shaving with no hair removal, found disadvantages for shaving only in observational studies [6–9] and as tendencies in one of two randomized studies [10,11]. They concluded that data gave some support to the claim that not shaving patients undergoing surgical procedures is preferable to preoperative shaving.

When shaving was compared with clipping, the authors found better supporting data in favor of clipping. They identified the best two of three randomized and two observational studies that found that clipping was associated with fewer SSIs compared with shaving [12–14]. They concluded that strong data indicated that clipping should be used instead of shaving if hair is removed preoperatively.

When shaving was compared with depilation, the authors found two randomized studies that failed to show differences between shaving and depilation [1]. Depilation was shown to be better than shaving in preventing SSIs in two observational studies [15,16]. The authors concluded that these data gave some strength to advocating that depilation should be used rather than shaving.

The authors found that moderate evidence exists to recommend removal of hair as close as possible to the time of the surgical procedure. Seropian and Reynolds showed a significantly increased risk for postoperative SSIs when patients were shaved more than 12 hours before surgery (ie, 12.4%) compared with patients shaved less than 2 hours before surgery (ie, 4.9%) [1]. Infection rates were doubled when hair removal by clipping was performed the evening before surgery (ie, 3.2%) in a randomized study of 1,013 patients [12]. The authors concluded that the evidence supporting hair removal close to surgery start is based on one randomized study for clipping and two observational studies for shaving.

The authors found only one observational study that addressed wet and dry shaving [17]. The study showed a nonsignificant doubling of infection rates after shaving when compared with electric clipping. The study was only designed to find general trends.

The author's assessment of this systematic literature review of preoperative hair removal is listed below:

- It is not strongly documented that hair removal results in a higher frequency of SSIs than no hair removal.
- Several randomized and observational studies with controls show that either wet or dry shaving the evening before the procedure results in a significantly higher infection rate that depilation or electric clipping.

- There are no convincing differences in the incidence of postoperative SSIs between electric clipping, depilation, or no hair removal.
- Hair removal with clippers should be performed as close as possible to the time of procedure.

The authors recommended that future research should be directed toward randomized trials of clipping or depilation versus no hair removal. They stated if observational studies are used, they should be contingent upon proper accounting for confounding factors (eg, age, sex, comorbidity, antibiotic prophylaxis, and type of surgery). In addition, studies would also require proper data analysis.

The second systemic review presented was published in 2005 by the Dutch Working Party on Infection Prevention (WIP) [3]. Their review of preoperative hair removal policies was conducted for similar reasons given by the authors of the previous review. Because the CDC guideline on this topic did not describe their evidence methods for its preoperative hair removal recommendations, the WIP conducted a systematic review of the literature. The comparisons addressed included the following: (1) no preoperative hair removal compared with preoperative hair removal, (2) hair removal the morning of surgery compared with removal the night before surgery, (3) hair removal by clipper versus razor, and (5) hair removal by clipper versus with cream.

The authors described strict selection criteria of preoperative hair removal studies of clean surgical procedures. They excluded trials of patients undergoing cranial neurosurgery. The selection criteria included studies in all languages that were planned as a randomized trial, quasirandomized trial, or systematic review of meta-analysis of randomized or quasirandomized trials; published as an article; involved hair that was removed by razor, clipper, or cream; involved hair that was removed the day before or the morning of surgery; and had sufficient data to calculate the risks of SSIs in both the treatment and control groups. Thirteen (13) abstracts were found that appeared to fulfill the selection criteria. However, after complete reading, only four trials were selected for review.

The following findings were reported for the various approaches. One eligible trial compared no preoperative hair removal with preoperative hair removal [12]. There were three arms to this study—no hair removal, hair removal by razor, and hair removal by cream. The time of hair removal was either the day before surgery or the day of surgery. The results favored no hair removal when compared with hair removal by razor. However, the results were not statistically significant. The authors did not pool the results for hair removal by razor and cream because of conflicting findings.

The comparison of hair removal the morning of surgery compared with the night before surgery was addressed in one eligible trial. There were four arms to this randomized trial of participants undergoing elective, major surgery: hair removal by razor and hair removal by clipper the morning before surgery, and hair removal the night before surgery by razor and by clipper. No difference was found between the groups when hair was removed by razor. Patients that had hair removal by clipper the morning of surgery had one third the risk of SSIs compared with patients that had hair removed the night before surgery. These were nearly statistically significant results. The data for hair removal by razor and clipper were not pooled because of inconsistent findings.

Comparison of preoperative hair removal by clipper and razor was addressed in two eligible trials. Participants undergoing elective inguinal herniorraphy were randomly assigned to 2 groups: hair removal by clipper or razor immediately before surgery [13]. The authors reported the pooled analysis resulted in a significant SSI risk reduction when hair was removed by clipper. The results of hair removal the night before surgery and the morning of surgery were combined because they were comparable. An SSI risk reduction of the pooled analyses was shown in favor of hair removal by clipper that was statistically significant.

Two eligible trials compared preoperative hair removal by cream with razor. Hair removal by cream the day before surgery or the day of surgery compared with hair removal by razor the day before surgery or the day of surgery showed results that favored hair removal by cream; although, the results were not statistically significant. The results of hair removal the morning of surgery and the night before surgery were not pooled because of conflicting findings. No eligible trials were found that compared preoperative hair removal by clipper with cream.

Although this systemic review identified four trials that met the established criteria of the authors, it was felt that the overall quality of the trials and the way in which they were reported were unsatisfactory. The authors felt that data from the trials were sparse and inconclusive that hair removal has any effect. Some evidence was shown that hair removal by clipper is superior to hair removal by razor.

The authors stated that the principal research design for a medical intervention, such as hair removal, is a randomized, controlled trial. They felt that the CDC's ranking system for its recommendations was too crude. The differences in susceptibility to bias of the various study designs (ie, randomized, controlled trials or observational studies) are not reflected in their classification system. As a result, the authors concluded that more evidence is warranted concerning the CDC's recommendations on hair removal policies than is really available.

The inconclusive evidence that hair removal affected the incidence of SSIs, as well as ward management issues when hair removal is recommended, led the WIP to recommend that hair removal not be performed preoperatively unless the hair at or around the incision site would interfere with the operation. The same rationale was given by WIP as a reason for them not to give a recommendation for time of hair removal. They recommended hair removal by clipper and stated that no eligible trials were found to compare hair removal by clipper with that by cream.

The authors concluded that large, randomized, controlled trials are needed to determine the optimal policy for preoperative removal of hair. They advised that studies be performed on clean surgical patients undergoing the same elective procedure where an incision is made in an area of considerable hair growth. All study participants should have hair removed at the same time when different methods are compared. Hair should be removed by the same method in all study participants when different removal times are compared.

The third systemic review of preoperative hair removal was published in March 2007 [4]. The authors reviewed the various methods of hair removal and recommendations by the CDC, the Norwegian Centre for Health Technology Assessment and the British Hospital Infection Society Working Party guidelines. The objective of this review, as stated by the authors, was to determine if routine preoperative hair removal results in fewer SSIs than not removing hair.

The authors described the study methods and the structured process of a systemic review, which they stated should be performed by using randomized, controlled trials that are assessed for quality. The search methods were described as thorough and exhaustive. Seven databases were used and additional articles were found through the search. Included in the review were 11 randomized, controlled trials that met the criteria of the authors. The trials were used to answer the following questions.

Does preoperative hair removal result in fewer surgical site infections than no hair removal?

Shaving compared with no hair removal—Two trials involving abdominal surgical procedures were used to answer this question [15,18]. The data analysis showed no statistically significant difference between hair removal and no hair removal using a razor. However, it was noted that these were not high-quality trials, and the sample size was too small to draw conclusions.

Depilatory cream compared with no hair removal—One trial involving abdominal surgery compared cream with no hair removal. The study did not provide details of randomization, allocation, and blinding methods. No statistically significant difference between the two groups was found. However, it was concluded that the sample size in this trial was also too small to draw conclusions.

Trials comparing clipping with no hair removal were not found by the authors.

What are the relative effects of shaving, clipping, and depilatory creams on surgical site infection?

Shaving compared with clipping to reduce SSIs—Three trials were included, which consisted of a total of 3193 predominantly clean procedures (hernia repair and cardiac surgery). Similar to other trials, full details of randomization, allocation, and blinding were not found. A statistically significant difference was shown for the likelihood of development of an SSI when shaving rather than clipping was performed before surgery.

Shaving compared with cream to reduce SSIs—The authors reviewed seven trials of variable quality in this category, involving 1213 patients [1,19–21]. It was shown by met-analysis that SSIs were more likely to develop in patients when shaved with a razor than having hair removed using a depilatory cream.

Clipping compared with cream to reduce SSIs—The authors stated that no trials were found that compared clipping with hair removal using a depilatory cream.

What is the effect on SSI rates of hair removal immediately before surgery compared with hair removal more than 4 hours before surgery?

Shaving the day of surgery compared with shaving 1 day preoperatively—One study involving 537 elective surgical procedures was identified by the authors [12]. No statistically significant difference between the groups relative to the risk of developing SSIs was found by meta-analysis. However, the authors stated that the sample size was too small to draw conclusions.

Clipping the day of surgery compared with clipping 1 day preoperatively—This comparison was found in one study involving 476 elective clean surgical procedures [12]. The SSI rate for those patients clipped 1 day preoperatively was 7.4% compared with 3.2% for those clipped on the day of surgery. These rates were not statistically different; however, the sample size was reported to be too small to draw conclusions.

No trials were found comparing depilation with cream on the day of surgery compared with clipping 1 day preoperatively. In addition, the authors reported that no trials were found that compared hair removal in different settings.

The authors concluded that because no trials were found that compared no hair removal and hair removal by clippers, it was not possible to make statements regarding hair removal versus no hair removal. As a result, the authors did not support the CDC recommendations nor those of the Hospital Infection Society, who strongly recommend that shaving should be avoided unless completely necessary. However, the findings of the Norwegian Centre for Health Technology Assessment is supported by the authors, which states that no strong evidence exists in favor or against preoperative hair removal.

The statistically significant finding that hair removal by clippers was associated with fewer SSIs than hair removal by razors, supports the recommendations of CDC and the Norwegian Health Technology Assessment. The review supported those recommendations.

No difference was found in clipping or shaving on the day of surgery compared with clipping or shaving 1 day preoperatively. It was noted that because these trials only involved 500 participants, not enough data were available to draw conclusions. Therefore, the authors stated that evidence found in this review does not support CDC recommendations or those of the Norwegian Health Technology Assessment, who advocate hair removal immediately before surgery.

Neurosurgical patient

Hair removal of the neurosurgical patient deserves special mention. Preoperative hair removal of the neurosurgical patient, which results in totally or partially shaved heads has been reported to stigmatize patients and cause psychologic problems [22]. Research has been performed to determine if not shaving the head of neurosurgical patients would increase the risk of infection. Kretschmer [23] reported results of a study of 215 cranial neurosurgical operations. One infection was identified giving a rate of 0.05%, which corresponded with their general infection rate of 0.6%, when hair was shaved. A study of 100 consecutive prospective nonrandomized neurosurgical procedures was performed of 90 pediatric patients aged 7 days to 16 years [24]. The children were divided into two groups: those who had hair shaved and those with no hair shaved. No significant difference was found in wound infection rates between the two arms. The authors concluded that no shaving was a good alternative to the traditional hair shaving approach, which allowed patients to enjoy the psychologic benefits of no disturbed body image. Iwami [22] evaluated 82 cranial surgery patients with the purpose to demonstrate methods and tips for cranial surgery without hair removal and evaluate postoperative infection rates. Superficial wound infections (2.4%) that were cured by antibiotic ointment developed in two patients. These and other articles [23,25] suggest that not performing preoperative hair removal does not increase the risk of SSI in the neurosurgical patient.

Survey of surgical attending staff

A short survey was conducted in a large teaching hospital to assess the current hair removal practices among surgical attending staff. Seventy-nine questionnaires were sent and 26 were returned with a response rate of 33%. Surgical services surveyed included cardiothoracic (30% response rate, 3 of 10); general surgery (29% response rate, 7 of 24); obstetrics/gynecology (25% response rate, 3 of 12); orthopedics (27% response rate, 6 of 22); neurosurgery (57% response rate, 4 of 7), and vascular (75% response rate, 3 of 4). The years of surgical practice ranged from 1 to 40, with and average of 16 years and median of 15 years.

The survey consisted of two practice questions. (1) "What do you base your hair removal practice on?" A choice of 5 responses was provided, to select all that applied, and one fill-in "other" choice was given. In response to this question, 41% of the responses (14 of 34) based their practice on common practices of others/peers, 26% (9 of 34) on CDC guidelines, 18% (6 of 34) on literature review of studies, 12% (4 of 34) on hospital policy/protocols, and 3% (1 of 34) fill-in response (personal preference). (2) "Which practice do you follow?" A choice of 5 responses was provided, to select all that applied. Fifty percent of the responses to this question (18 of 36) were hair removal by clipper directly before surgery, 31% of responses (11 of 36) were no hair removal unless hair at or around the site would interfere with the operation, and 19% (7 of 36) chose hair removal by razor directly before surgery. The last question was a test of knowledge regarding the preferred method of hair removal recommended by the CDC. Forty-three percent (15 of 35) and 37% (13 of 35), respectively, chose the correct response of hair removal by clippers and no hair removal unless hair was at or around the incision site. Hair removal by razor directly before surgery was selected by 14% (5 of 35). Of note, those responders were from the obstetrics/gynecology surgeons (2), neurosurgeons (1), and orthopedic surgeons (2). Two responders (6%) stated they did not know CDC's recommendation for hair removal.

Summary

The above three systematic literature reviews on preoperative hair removal had similar findings (Table 1). Although there are numerous published articles on this subject, findings of many were inconclusive because of unsatisfactory study design ranging from issues with randomization methods, small number of study participants, and the use of historical controls and observational studies versus randomized controlled trials. There was insufficient evidence to state whether hair removal has any impact on SSIs. In addition, all of the reviews concluded that if hair removal is performed before surgery, clipping and depilatory creams result in fewer SSIs than shaving. The need for more research with large, well-designed, randomized, controlled trials or observational studies was recommended to establish the best practice for preoperative hair removal. The CDC 1999 preoperative hair removal recommendations are consistent with the literature. However, the strongly recommended, category IA suggests more evidence than is really available.

Table 1
Systematic literature review

Article reference	No. of studies	Type	Findings
Kjonniksen, et al [2]	120	Randomized; observational	Moderate evidence supports hair removal is close to time of operative procedure. No convincing differences in the incidence of SSIs between electric clippers, depilation, or no hair removal. More research directed toward randomized trials of clipping or depilation versus no hair removal is needed
Niel-Weiss, et al [3]	4	Randomized; quasi-randomized or systematic review of meta-analysis	Results favored no hair removal when compared with hair removal by razor. SSI risk reduction when hair removed by clippers. Large randomized, controlled trials needed to determine best policy for preoperative hair removal.
Tanner J, et al [4]	11	Randomized control trials	Hair removal by clippers was associated with fewer SSIs than hair removed by razor.

Literature on preoperative hair removal of the neurosurgical patient has shown that SSIs are not increased when no hair removal is performed. When hair is not removed, the surgical closing will get more tedious, will require additional training, and will prolong the procedure. However, this option is available for female patients or children who may have strong psychologic issues with hair removal during neurosurgical procedures.

The results of the preoperative hair removal survey suggest that many of the 26 surgeons who responded based their hair removal protocol on common practice of their peers. The survey disclosed noncompliance with clipping-only protocols on several services. A neurosurgeon, in practice for 40 years, selected hair removal by razor directly before surgery as his hair removal practice. Hair removal by razor was also identified in three obstetrics/gynecology and three orthopedic surgeon responses. Eighty percent of the surgeon responses correctly identified the CDC recommendation for preoperative hair removal. Several surgeons had written comments regarding the issue of dressing placement and removal when hair is not removed.

To answer the opening question: based on this review, either practice (hair removal by clipping directly before surgery or no hair removal) is acceptable. The literature contains no convincing differences between electric clipping, depilation, or no hair removal in the incidence of postoperative SSIs. There are multifactorial strategies that impact the occurrence of surgical site infections. It is essential that each factor be integrated into a bundle strategy in an attempt to provide an infection-free outcome for the patient.

References

[1] Seropian R, Reynolds BM. Wound infection after preoperative depilatory vs. razor prep. Am J Surg 1971;121:251–4.

[2] Kjonniksen I, Andersen BM, et al. Preoperative hair removal—a systematic review. AORN J 2002;75(5):928–40.

[3] Niel-Weiss BS, Willie JC, et al. Hair removal policies in clean surgery: a systematic review of randomized controlled trials. Infect Control Hosp Epidemiol 2005;26(12):923–8.

[4] Tanner J, Moncaster K, et al. Preoperative hair removal: a systematic review. J Perioper Pract 2007;17(3):118–31.

[5] Mangram AJ, Horan TC, et al. CDC Guideline for Prevention of surgical site infection. Infect Control Hosp Epidemiol 1999;20:250–78.

[6] Moro ML, et al. Risk factors for surgical wound infections in clean surgery: a multicenter study. Ann Ital Chir 1996;67:13–9.

[7] Morgan MA, Piatt JH Jr. Shaving of the scalp may increase the rate of infection in CSF shunt surgery. Pediatr Neurosurg 1997;26:180–4.

[8] Cruse PJ, Ford R. The epidemiology of wound infection: a 10 year prospective study of 62,939 wounds. Surg Clin North Am 1980;60:27–40.

[9] Winston KR. Hair and neurosurgery. Neurosurgery 1992;31:320–9.

[10] Ko W, Lazenby WD, Zelano JA, et al. Effects of shaving methods and intraoperative irrigation on suppurative mediastinitis after bypass operations. Ann Thorac Surg 1992;53:301–5.

[11] Hoe NY, Nambiar R. Is preoperative shaving really necessary? Ann Acad Med Singapore 1985;14: 700–4.

[12] Alexander W, et al. The influence of hair-removal methods on wound infections. Arch Surg 1983;118: 347–52.

[13] Balthazar ER, Colt JD, Nichols RL. Preoperative hair removal: a random prospective study of shaving versus clipping. South Med J 1982;75:799–801.

[14] Sellick JA Jr, Stelmach M, Mylotte JM. Surveillance of surgical wound infections following open heart surgery. Infect Control Hosp Epidemiol 1991;12: 591–6.

[15] Court-Brown CM. Preoperative skin depilation and its effect on post-operative wound infections. J R Coll Surg Edinb 1981;26:238–41.

[16] Thur de Koos P, McComas B. Shaving versus skin depilatory cream for preoperative skin preparation: a prospective study of wound infection rates. Am J Surg 1983;145:377–8.

[17] Zentner J, Gilsbach J, Daschner F. Incidence of wound infection in patients undergoing craniotomy: influence of type of shaving. Acta Neurochir (Wien) 1987;75:79–82.

[18] Rojanapirom S, Danchaivijitr S. Preoperative shaving and wound infection in appendectomy. J Med Assoc Thai 1992;75(2):20–3.

[19] Breiting V, Helberg S. Chemical depilation as an alternative to shaving. Ugeskrift fur Laeger 1981; 143:1646–7 [in Danish].

[20] Powis SJA, Waterworth T, Arkell D. Preoperative skin preparation: clinical evaluation of depilatory cream. Br Med J 1976;2:1166–8.

[21] Thorup J, Fischer A, Lindenberg S, et al. Chemical depilation versus shaving. Ugeskrift fur Laeger 1985;21(13):1108–10.

[22] Iwami K, Takagi T, Arima T, et al. [Cranial surgery without shaving: practice and results in our hospital]. No Shinkei Geka 2006;34(9):901–5 [in Japanese].

[23] Kretschmer T, Braun V, et al. Neurosurgery without shaving: indications and results. Br J Neurosurg 2000;14(4):341–4.

[24] Tang K, Yeh JS. The influence of hair shave on the infection rate in neurosurgery: a prospective study. Pediatr Neurosurg 2001;35(1):13–7.

[25] Bekar A, Korfali E, Dogan S, et al. The effect of hair removal on infection after cranial surgery. Acta Neurochir (Wien) 2001;143(6):533–6.

ELSEVIER
SAUNDERS

Perioperative Nursing Clinics 3 (2008) 115–120

PERIOPERATIVE
NURSING
CLINICS

Preparing for the Patient Who Has Prion Disease

Cynthia Spry, RN, MA, MSN, CNOR

350 Bleecker Street, Apartment 4J, New York, NY 10014, USA

The mention of Creutzfeldt-Jakob (CJD) disease can be cause for apprehension in those responsible for the patients and/or for those responsible for cleaning, disinfecting, or sterilizing devices, including surgical instruments, used on a known or suspected patient with this disease. Although CJD has been discussed in the medical literature for many years, it is only in the last 10 or so years that it has become a "hot topic." The identification of a variant form of the disease, that first became evident in the United Kingdom in 1996, brought with it predictions for an emerging epidemic that would result in the death of thousands [1]. Although that prediction did not become reality, both classical CJD and the new variant form remain topics of significant interest.

CJD and the variant form of CJD, new variant CJD (nvCJD), are two of a number of fatal transmissible spongiform encephalopathies (TSEs). Other TSEs in humans are Gerstmann-Straussler-Scheinker syndrome (GSS), fatal familiar insomnia (FFI), sporadic familial insomnia, kuru, and Alper's syndrome. In animals, TSE diseases include scrapie in goats and sheep, chronic wasting disease in mule deer and elk, transmissible mink encephalopathy (TME), feline spongiform encephalopathy in cats, and bovine spongiform encephalopathy (BSE) in cattle. The latter is commonly known as *mad cow disease*.

TSEs are thought to be caused by a prion, a proteinaceous particle. Prions are made from proteins that normally are found in the central nervous system. The difference is that the prion protein has a different structure and is resistant to enzymes within the body that break down normal proteins. It is not known what causes normal protein to become abnormal and, in turn, infectious. Prions contain no DNA or RNA and replicate by converting normal protein into aberrant protein. Prion diseases are always fatal, and prions are resistant to inactivation.

Because TSEs have a lengthy incubation period, it was originally thought that a "slow virus" was the cause. However, Stanley Prusiner is credited with the discovery of prions and received the Nobel Prize in 1997 for his work [2]. As a result, it is believed that prions are responsible for TSEs. Interestingly, however, a 2007 paper by Yale neuropathologist, Laura Manduelidis, et al, reports the discovery of a responsible virus [3]. It should be noted that much is not known about prions, research is ongoing, and recommendations for care of the patient and devices used on that patient are evolving and sometimes conflicting.

Prions aggregate within the central nervous system forming plaques known as "amyloids." Amyloids disrupt cell function, cause cell death, and cause vacuoles or holes to occur within brain tissue giving it a spongy appearance, hence the term "spongiform."

TSEs, also known as prion diseases, illicit no immune response. They are degenerative brain diseases for which there is no known cure, and although the symptoms vary among prion diseases, all are fatal neurologic diseases. Symptoms typically include neurologic deficits such as ataxia, convulsions, dementia, and personality changes.

GSS is extremely rare with the incidence estimated to be somewhere between one in a billion [4]. Symptoms include disarthria, ataxia, and dementia.

FFI is an inherited disease and has been found in only 40 families worldwide [5]. Symptoms include hallucinations, insomnia, and subsequent weight loss followed by dementia and finally mutism.

E-mail address: Cynthia350@gmail.com

Kuru is restricted to the Fore tribe in the highlands of Papua, New Guinea. The word "kuru" means "trembling with fear." Funeral practices in the Fore tribe included ritualistic cooking and eating of the deceased. The brain, the most infectious organ, was given to the closest relatives, and, as a result, whole families and much of the tribe died. Cannibalism has all but disappeared, and kuru is almost nonexistent today. It is not known how kuru originated, but it is suspected that consumption of the meat of an animal, perhaps a sheep, with a prion disease may have been the origin [6].

CJD, the most common prion disease, manifests itself with symptoms of rapidly progressive dementia. Onset is insidious. Sensory deficits, cognitive changes, memory loss, and ataxia are among the first symptoms. These are followed by myoclonus and incapacitation. In the final stages the patient is usually mute and immobile. The incidence of classic CJD worldwide is approximately one in one million [7]. There is no screening assay that can detect the prion protein in asymptomatic individuals. CJD is suspected when a patient exhibits rapidly progressive dementia with accompanying myoclonus. Diagnosis most often is made in individuals over 55 years with the median age of 68 at time of death, which occurs within less than 1 year after diagnosis. According to the Centers for Disease Control (CDC), the United States has reported less than 300 cases per year [8]. Diagnosis is made principally on the basis of clinical symptoms and neuropathologic examination. A lumbar puncture may be performed to eliminate other possible causes, but it cannot confirm CJD. Electroencephalographic changes include sharp triphasic spikes; however, a definitive diagnosis can only be made through neuropathologic examination, eg, examination of brain tissue. Because brain biopsy on suspected CJD patients is not routine and is not recommended, except to make a diagnosis of a treatable disease, the practitioner caring for the patient or handling the devices used on that patient must take specific precautions on all suspected as well as known CDJ patients.

There are several categories of classic CJD: Sporadic, representing approximately 85% to 90% of all cases; familial, representing 10% of cases; and iatrogenic, representing 10% of cases. Iatrogenic incidence involves direct contact with high-risk tissue. The World Health Organization (WHO) estimates 313 CJD cases have occurred as a result of iatric incidence; injection of pituitary growth hormone made from human cadavers who died of CJD (a practice stopped in 1985 and replaced by recombinant growth hormone [167 cases]); implantation of contaminated grafts, ie, cornea (3 cases) or dura mater (136 cases); stereotactic electrodes (2 cases); and transmission from contaminated neurosurgical instruments (5 cases) [9]. Since 1974 there have been no further incidences of transmission via reprocessed surgical instruments. There have been no reported incidences of nvCJD transmission associated with reprocessed surgical instruments. There have, however, been three reported cases of nvCJD transmission from blood transfusions, suggesting transmission via an nvCJD-infected donor [10]. Because of the lengthy incubation period for nvCDJ the number of patients who may contract the disease from blood transfusions is not known. The United Kingdom and the United States, among other countries, have instituted policies prohibiting blood donations from persons with risk factors for nvCDJ.

New variant CJD is associated with consumption of beef from cattle infected with BSE. The minimum infectious dose is unknown. The first sign of an epidemic of BSE was identified in November 1986 in the United Kingdom when scientists recognized a new neurologic disease in cattle. Between 1986 and 2002 181,376 cases were identified. Ten years later in 1996 the first case of nvCDJ was recognized, and it is therefore assumed that the incubation period is at least 10 years. As of September 2007, 170 people in the United Kingdom and 11 countries outside the United Kingdom but who had been in the United Kingdom or eaten imported beef, have died of nvCJD as a result of consuming prion-contaminated beef. It is estimated that between 460,000 and 482,000 infected cattle entered the food chain before controls were put in place to prevent the infection in cattle. The source of BSE was from contaminated feed. Cattle are normally herbivores, but in industrial cattle farming protein supplements are also provided. Until 1989 cattle were fed the remains of other cattle and sheep in the form of bone meal. In addition, the temperature for rendering cattle had been reduced and prions can withstand high temperatures. It is probable that infected animals were included in the preparation of supplemental bone meal. New food chain controls were introduced in 1989 and roughly 4.4 million cattle were slaughtered as a precaution. As a result, the incidence of BSE has declined to zero, and the number of patients with nvCJD is less than five per year. Because of the lengthy incubation period, the number of people who will eventually have nvCJD is as yet unknown [11].

The symptoms of nvCJD and the incubation period differ from classical CJD. The median age at death is 28, with death occurring approximately 5 months after diagnosis. Presenting symptoms are sensory and psychiatric disturbances and painful sensations like pricks of pins and needles. Neurologic symptoms are demonstrated later on in the disease process [8].

Prion diseases are not transmitted person to person. In addition to direct exposure to contaminated growth hormone, brain, or eye tissue, CJD has been transmitted as a result of exposure to infectious prion-contaminated surgical instruments. Five cases are attributed to contaminated neurosurgical instruments and two to contaminated stereotactic depth electrodes. The electrodes had been implanted in a known CJD patient then processed in 70% alcohol and exposed to formaldehyde vapor and stored. Two years later they were implanted into a chimpanzee that then contracted CJD. The neurosurgical instruments were cleaned with soap and water and exposed to dry heat. Exposure time and temperature are not known. These iatrogenic cases all occurred between 1953 and 1976 when instrument processing procedures were quite different from and less stringent than procedures used today. It is interesting to note that there are no documented cases of iatrogenic prion disease resulting from contaminated instruments even in the face of the recent epidemic of nvCDJ in the United Kingdom. According to Rutala and Weber, the reason is probably because, with the exception of brain and neural tissue, transmission is ineffective and also because of effective instrument processing protocols and procedures [7].

As a result of the UK epidemic of BSE and subsequent nvCJD, a number of agencies and professional societies responsible for writing guidelines identified protocols for processing surgical instruments used on patients exposed to known or suspected CJD patients. The WHO, the Association of periOperative Registered Nurses and Advisory Committee on Dangerous Pathogens and Spongiform Encephalopathy are three such organizations. In addition, in June 2001 the Joint Commission (JCAHO) issued a sentinel alert after it received reports of two separate incidences in accredited hospitals in which a total of 14 patients may have been exposed to instruments used during brain surgery on patients who had CJD. The sentinel alert recommended that hospitals establish policies for (1) the disinfection or disposal of instruments used in neurosurgery in general and when CJD is suspected or confirmed and (2) the

quarantine of such surgical instruments until a clear diagnosis is made [12].

The WHO guidelines include recommendations for decontamination of surgical instruments by several methods, one of which is immersion in sodium hydroxide and then autoclaving in a steam sterilizer. This particular recommendation was addressed by sterilizer manufacturers who said this practice can result in damaging the autoclave and voiding its warranty. In addition, instrument processing personnel were concerned about the possibility of exposure to toxic fumes [13]. Recommendations and guidelines do vary between organizations and countries. Many hospitals, in particular the instrument processing departments, have struggled to be compliant with JCAHO, WHO, and other guidelines.

Fear of CJD disease in the midst of the BSE epidemic led to inconsistent care of the patient. Excessive and unnecessary use of gowns, gloves, masks, and dedicated medical equipment was practiced in a number of institutions. There is, however, no evidence that health care workers are at increased occupational risk for CJD or that CJD is transmitted easily, and as science replaced fear, a more rational approach to patient care evolved.

The chain of infection transmission includes an infectious agent, a reservoir, a portal of exit, mode of transmission, portal of entry, and a susceptible host. All of these must be present for infection to occur. In the case of CJD, unless an invasive procedure is performed on the patient there is no portal of exit and no mode of transmission. Therefore, care of the CDJ patient should mimic the care given to any patient with symptoms of sensory impairment, discomfort, and dementia. The symptoms should dictate care. As the patient becomes decreasingly debilitated, the patient will become highly dependent and will increasingly need assistance. There is no need to place the patient in isolation; a private room is not necessary for other than compassionate reasons, and there is no need for dedicated medical equipment. Personal protective equipment protocols should reflect standard precautions. This holds true for the operating room as well. When preparing the operating room or a patient room to receive a known or suspected CJD patient, there is no need to remove equipment from the room or practice precautions other than standard precautions. No special precautions are necessary for body fluids or linen. Medical waste from a known or suspected CJD patient should be handled in the same manner as other regulated waste, ie, according to state regulatory requirements. Extreme approaches to terminal cleaning and disinfecting of a room occupied by a CJD patient are unnecessary as well.

Transmission occurs by direct tissue to tissue contact or indirect contact of a contaminated item to tissue. Examples of direct tissue contact include blood transfusion and cornea transplant. Examples of indirect contact include surgical instruments that contact prion-contaminated tissue, are not properly processed, and subsequently used on another patient undergoing neurosurgery.

Although TSEs are not transmissible from person to person, they can be transmitted during invasive procedures if the devices used are contaminated with prions and inadequately reprocessed. Prions are resistant to the routine sterilization cycles used in hospitals today, and special procedures must be practiced when reprocessing known or suspected prion-contaminated surgical instruments.

It is important to note that the research results on inactivation of prions have been inconsistent. This is because research test methods, prion concentrations, test tissue, test animals, and sterilization cycle parameters have not been consistent. What is agreed on, however, is that prions are resistant to the routine sterilization cycles used in hospitals. Prions are resistant to chemicals—alcohols, detergents, glutaraldehyde, peracetic acid, hydrogen peroxide, iodophors, and phenolics; gases—ethylene oxide, formaldehyde; physical methods—boiling, dry heat, ionizing radiation, and ultraviolet and conventional steam sterilization cycles.

A rationale approach to the care of instruments used on a known or suspected CDJ patient involves first determining the risk of transmission. The patient, the tissue, and the device must all be assessed. Assessment should be implemented to determine whether the patient is a high-risk patient, whether the patient will undergo an invasive procedure that involves contact with high-risk tissue, and finally whether the device(s) are critical devices. A critical device is defined as a device that is used to penetrate mucous membranes or that contacts a normally sterile area of the body. Critical devices require sterilization [14].

Is the patient a high-risk patient (possible or known CJD patient)?

- Confirmed diagnosis
- Symptoms suggestive of CDJ—rapidly progressive degenerative neurologic disorder of unknown origin
- Symptoms suggestive of CJD coupled with consumption of beef in the United Kingdom 1986–1990

- Family history of CJD
- Recipient of dura mater
- Recipient of growth hormone before 1985
- Recipient of cornea transplant

Is the tissue high-risk tissue?
- High-risk tissue (tissue with a high prion load)—brain, spinal cord, and eye
- Low infectivity—cerebrospinal fluid, kidney, liver, lung, lymph nodes/spleen

Will critical devices be used to treat this patient?

- Devices, eg, surgical instruments used in treatment/surgery that involve contact with high-risk tissue [15].

All three of these factors; high-risk patient, high-risk tissue, and critical device must be present to constitute the need for special instrument processing protocols. Written protocols should be in place for obtaining suitable instruments and equipment (single use may be best), handling, storage, quarantine, cleaning, sterilization, and disposal.

Studies indicate that cleaning followed by steam sterilization using an extended cycle is effective, and this is how most hospitals today process known or suspected prion-contaminated instruments. Recent studies indicate that hydrogen peroxide gas plasma, peracetic acid, and ozone sterilization after cleaning with an alkaline detergent may be effective as well. Recommendations for application using these technologies are evolving and may be forthcoming shortly.

Decontamination of contaminated medical devices that contact high-risk tissue requires special procedures as follows:

- Use disposable surgical instruments if possible [16].
- Do not use flash sterilization.
- Devices that are constructed so as to be easily and effectively cleaned should be cleaned and then steam sterilized at 134°C for ≥18 minutes in a prevacuum sterilizer or at 121°C to 132°C for 1 hour in a gravity-displacement sterilizer.
- Devices that are impossible to clean should be discarded.
- Devices that are difficult to clean may be discarded or may be placed in a container of liquid, eg, water or saline, to retard adherence of debris, then removed from the liquid then initially decontaminated by steam sterilization at 134°C for 18 minutes in a prevacuum sterilizer or at 121°C to 132°C for 1 hour in a gravity-displacement sterilizer; or by soaking the

device in 1normal (N) NaOH for 1 hour. The device is then cleaned, wrapped, and terminally sterilized by conventional means [7]. Serrations, lumens, crevices, ratchets, and multi joints that cannot be disassembled are particularly difficult to clean.

- JCAHO recommends quarantine of the instruments until a definitive diagnosis is made.

Decontamination of devices contaminated with low-risk or no-risk tissue may be cleaned and disinfected or sterilized using conventional protocols for instrument processing.

Decontamination of noncritical environmental surfaces, such as laboratory surfaces, that come in contact with brain tissue from a high-risk CJD patient, should be cleaned with a detergent and then spot-decontaminated with 5,000 ppm sodium hypochlorite. Noncritical equipment contaminated with high-risk tissue should be cleaned and then disinfected with 5,000 ppm sodium hypochlorite or 1N NaOH depending on material compatibility [17].

A most important implementation in planning the care of the patient with a prion disease is communication. When a known or suspected prion disease patient is scheduled for surgery, the operating room staff must be notified of the diagnosis. Infection control and central processing departments must also be notified. When a specimen is involved, laboratory/pathology personnel must be informed. Advance notification of admission should be provided to any receiving unit. Advance notice provides an opportunity for review of the mechanism of CJD transmission, circumstances when additional precautions are necessary, and provides time to allay any unnecessary fears surrounding the care of the patient.

Other preparatory activities:

- Develop policies for patient assessment relative to CJD.
- Educate all staff who may be affected.
- Consider scheduling surgery at the end of the day when there are fewer people around and the OR is often less hectic.
- If possible, do not use relief personnel during the surgical procedure—avoid opportunity for missed communication.
- Minimize number of personnel involved in the procedure.
- Use disposable surgical instruments/devices when possible.

- Where possible, manual rather than power drills and equipment should be used because power tools are often difficult to clean.
- Use instruments that are functional but at the end of their life cycle and dispose after use.
- Keep number of items used in surgery to the minimum number and type needed.
- Implement a single flow of instruments, eg, instruments are retrieved from back table for use and then returned to Mayo stand, which allows for identification of instruments actually used in surgery.
- Implement an instrument tracking system that allows every device to be tracked to the patient, the procedure, date of procedure, and surgeon.
- Implement a system to tag items or sets that have been exposed to high-risk tissue so as to alert instrument processing personnel.
- Implement a system to process instruments as soon as possible after surgery to minimize or prevent adherence of blood, tissue, or body fluid to the instrument.

Research into inactivation of prions is ongoing and as such recommendations for instrument processing are evolving. Personnel responsible for instrument processing should remain current by checking with health care organizations and agencies such as the Association for Professionals in Infection Control (APIC) and the CDC for the most up-to-date guidelines.

There is no epidemiologic evidence that links CDJ transmission to disposal of waste when current medical waste practices are implemented and no additional protocols are necessary. Regulated medical waste should be managed according to state regulations. No special precautions are required for disposal of body fluids.

Disposable drapes should be used and discarded into infectious waste containers. Reusable drapes should be processed according to routine protocols.

Specimens should be marked with a biohazard label and the words "suspected CJD."

Although there is no documented case of TSE transmission from occupational exposure, the following are recommendations from WHO.

- Contamination of unbroken skin with internal body fluids or tissues: wash with detergent and abundant quantities of warm water (avoid scrubbing), rinse, and dry. Brief exposure (1 minute, to 0.1 N NaOH or a 1:10 dilution of bleach) can be considered for maximum safety.

- Needle sticks or lacerations: gently encourage bleeding; wash with warm soapy water, rinse, dry, and cover with a waterproof dressing.
- Splashes into the eye or mouth: irrigate with either saline (eye) or tap water (mouth) [18].

CDJ and nvCJD are fatal diseases caused by prions. Prions are resistant to inactivation using routine hospital decontamination, disinfection, and sterilization protocols. There is no documentation of transmission to health care workers through occupational accident or injury. Iatric transmission has occurred through dura mater transplantation, cornea transplant, injection of pituitary growth hormone and contaminated surgical instruments/devices. Since the early 1970s there have been no documented cases of transmission of either CJD or nvCJD. However, the possibility for transmission from contaminated surgical instruments is a possibility. Therefore, health care workers must assess the patient, nature of any intended invasive procedure, and the devices that will be used. When a high-risk patient undergoes surgery involving contact with high-risk tissue special procedures must be implemented to process the instruments so as to make them safe for the next patient. Research on prion inactivation is ongoing, and health care personnel should consult the recent literature when preparing for the patient with prion disease.

References

[1] Naik G. Mad-Cow in the U.K. is less than feared. The Wall Street Journal January 12, 2004.
[2] Prusiner S. Prions. Available at: http://www.nobelprize.org/nobel_prizes/medicine/laureates. Accessed September 20, 2007.
[3] Manuelidis L, Yu Z, Barquero N, et al. Cells infected with scrapie and Creutzfeldt-Jakob disease agents produce intracellular 25-nm virus-like particles. Proceedings of the National Academy of Science of the USA 2007;104(6):1965–70.
[4] Association for the Advancement of Medical Instrumentation (AAMI). Annex C processing CJD contaminated patient care equipment and environmental surfaces. In: Comprehensive guide to steam sterility and sterility assurance in health care facilities. Arlington (VA): AAMI; 2006. p. 127.
[5] Fatal familial insomnia. Available at: http://en.wikipedia.org/wiki/Fatal_familial_insomnia. Accessed September 17, 2007.
[6] Kuru disease. In: Wikipedia. Available at: http://en.wikipedia.org/wiki/Kuru_%28disease%29. Accessed September 17, 2007.
[7] Rutala WA, Weber DJ. Creutzfeldt-Jakob disease: recommendations for disinfection and sterilization. Clin Infect Dis 2001;32:1348–56.
[8] CJD (Creutzfeldt-Jakob Disease, Classic). Available at: http://www.cdc.gov/ncidod/dvrd/cjd/. Accessed September 20, 2007.
[9] World Health Organization (WHO). WHO guidelines on transmissible spongiform encephalopathy in relation to biological and pharmaceutical products. Available at: http://whqlibdoc.who.int/hq/2003/a85721.pdf. Accessed September 28, 2007. p. 2.
[10] BBC News. Third vCJD "blood case" diagnosed. February 9, 2006. Available at: http://news.bbc.co.uk/1/hi/helath/4696522. Accessed September 19, 2007.
[11] Bovine spongiform encephalopathy. In: Wikipedia. Available at: http://en.wikipedia.org/wiki/Bovine_spongiform_encephalopathy. Accessed September 19, 2007.
[12] The Joint Commission. Sentinel event alert: exposure to Creutzfeldt-Jakob disease. 2001;(20). Available at: http://www.jointcommission.org/SentinalEventsAlert/sea_20.htm. Accessed September 20, 2007.
[13] Favero M, Bond W. Chemical disinfection and antisepsis in the hospital. In: Favero M, Bond W, editors. Chemical disinfection, sterilization, and preservation. Philadelphia: Lippincott Williams & Wilkins; 2001.
[14] Fogg D. Creutzfeldt-Jakob disease. AORN J 2001; 74(3):726–9.
[15] WHO, Infection control guidelines for transmissible spongiform encephalopathies Report of WHO consultation. March; 1999. p. 4.
[16] WHO. 1999. p. 6.
[17] AAMI.P. 130.
[18] WHO. 1999. p. 10.

ELSEVIER
SAUNDERS

Perioperative Nursing Clinics 3 (2008) 121–126

PERIOPERATIVE
NURSING
CLINICS

Flash Sterilization Revisited

Mary Ann Magerl, RN, MA, CIC

Infection Control Department, Westchester Medical Center, 18 Massachusetts Drive, Valhalla, NY 12550, USA

Incredibly, surgical procedures were once conducted in open areas with bare hands. We have come a long way. Now strict requirements are in place for spaces used to perform surgery and the instruments and trays used in any surgical procedure must now be subjected to a cleaning, disinfection, or sterilization process. The system of flash sterilization was developed so that a surgical procedure already in progress would not need to be extended for a lengthy period to reprocess an instrument that had inadvertently been contaminated and was needed to complete the procedure.

The Association for the Advancement of Medical Instrumentation (AAMI) defines flash sterilization as "the process designated for the steam sterilization of patient-care items for immediate use." Flash sterilization is not recommended as a routine method of sterilization [1]. With flash sterilization, the exposure time to the steam is abbreviated in gravity steam sterilizers. So that the steam may have unrestricted access to the instruments, the instruments are not wrapped and no container systems are used [2]. This method is used when there is a need to sterilize items under emergency situations. An emergency may be defined as an uneventful drop of the instrument from the sterile field or the inadvertent contamination of an instrument due to contact with an unsterile surface or individual. Flash sterilization is not intended to be used as a convenient method of inventory control or as a convenience to avoid a trip to the instrument storage room. Flash sterilization is not an acceptable method of sterilization for implantable devices [1]. Biological indicators results developed for flash sterilization can be provided in 1 hour. Even so, flash sterilization is not recommended for routine use

for several reasons, such as the absence of protective packaging after sterilization, the possibility for contamination of processed items during transportation, and the use of minimal sterilization cycle parameters (ie, time, temperature, pressure) [1].

When using the flash sterilization process, applicable protocols must be followed. They include cleaning, decontaminating, inspecting, correctly arranging instruments in the correct container or tray, and placing instruments close to where they will be used. An operator should not need to go a great distance to deliver the sterilized instrument to the sterile field. Because of the lack of drying time, flash sterilized instruments are wet when the cycle is completed and should not be stored [2].

The three basic methods of sterilization by steam are gravity displacement, prevacuum steam, and steam-flush/pressure pulse. Sterilizer manufacturers generally offer products that employ a combination of gravity and prevacuum methods. Flash sterilization usually is achieved by the gravity method, because the use of other methods requires additional parameter testing [3]. Recommendations for flash sterilization come from two sources. The first is the Association of periOperative Registered Nurses (AORN) and the second is AAMI. The groups have similar recommendations focusing on standard protocols, the mechanical aspects of practice, the types of biological indicators required, and physical parameters.

Association of periOperative Registered Nurses recommended practice

AORN recommendations for practice, developed by the Recommended Practice Committee and approved by the AORN board of directors, address flash sterilization [4]. The recommendations note that flash sterilization should only be used in selected clinical situations and in

E-mail address: magerlm@wcmc.com

a controlled manner. Flash sterilization should be done using a minimum number of procedures and only under the following conditions:

- Manufacturer's written guidelines are available.
- Instruments are taken apart and thoroughly cleaned, which includes the removal of soil, blood, fats, and any other substances, before flash sterilization.
- The cleaning solution is flushed through all lumens and rinsed completely.
- Instruments are placed in such a manner that permits the steam to contact all parts of the instruments.
- All physical obstacles are removed before the sterile instruments are transported to a sterile field.
- Documentation is completed to permit the tracking of any flashed item to the individual patient.

AORN recommendations further state that flash sterilization may be used when insufficient time is available to process the instruments in the preferred fashion. However, flash sterilization should not be used as a substitute for insufficient instrumentation. Given the hectic pace in the operative arena and the frantic rush to resterilize a contaminated instrument needed for the procedure, it is easy to for individuals to skip one or more steps in the reprocessing process—cleaning, inspecting, and then subjecting to the flash sterilization process. It is imperative that all the steps be completed.

Prior to any flash sterilization, instruments must be cleaned and dried to ensure that the proper decontamination has removed any blood-borne pathogen, dirt, debris, and protein materials. Cleaning is the first step in decontamination. Failure to complete the appropriate cleaning will lead to failure of the sterilization process and may result in the transmission of infectious agents. The use of packaging and wrapping is not recommended when items are flash sterilized unless there is a specific recommendation by the sterilizer or instrument manufacturer.

Because packaging and wrapping should not be used in the flash sterilization process, special handling of unwrapped packages is needed during transportation to the point of use. This means procedures must be put in place to ensure that unsterile surfaces are not touched and that the flash sterilized item is aseptically delivered to the sterile field or removed from the container by a scrubbed member of the surgical team. Manufacturers offer specialized flash sterilization containers. These may serve to decrease the risk of contamination during the transport process after completion of flash sterilization. The manufacturer's guidelines must be used to ensure that these containers effectively perform the task. Additionally these containers need to be cleaned and stored between use, according to each manufacturer's guidelines.

Flash sterilization should not be used for implantable devices. Perioperative managers must develop and implement prudent policies and procedures, protocols, and a plan to diminish the need to flash-sterilize instruments, including implants. The plan should consist of careful checking and assessing instrument needs before a procedure. First, the need for an implant should be determined. Second, if an implant is needed, the inventory of sterile implants should be checked before scheduling and sterilizing the implants well in advance of the procedure. A biological indicator needs to be run with the load and the implant quarantined until the results of the biological indicator are known. In the event of an emergency and flash sterilization is unavoidable, a rapid-action biological should be used with a class V chemical integrator. The implant may be released for immediate use once the rapid-action indicator provides a negative result. Remember, if the implant is not used, it may not be stored as sterile. If the biological indicator is later determined to be positive, the surgeon should be notified as soon as possible.

Any time flash sterilization is being done, it must be monitored to ensure that all of the sterilization parameters are achieved. The physical parameters that should be monitored are time and temperature. The operator should ensure that parameters are met and documented before taking the sterile item to the operative field. Monitoring devices made specifically for flash sterilizers should be used according to the manufacturer's written instructions. There should be a monitoring device with each flash sterilization process. The device will demonstrate that conditions for sterilization have been met. Typical flash sterilization parameters include:

For high-speed gravity-displacement sterilizers: 3-minute cycle for metal or nonporous items with an exposure temperature of 270° F to 275° F (132°–135° C) and a drying time of up to 1 minute. For mixed items, metal items with lumens, porous items, and complex devices, such as powered instruments, a 10-minute cycle with an exposure temperature of 270° F to 275° F (132°–135° C) and a drying time of up to 1 minute. The manufacturer's recommendations for the applicable parameters must be followed for complex devices.

For pulse gravity sterilizers: Manufacturer's recommendations must be followed.

For prevacuum sterilizers: 3 minute cycle with an exposure temperature of 270°–275° F (132°–135° C) for metal or nonporous items only (ie, no lumens); 4 minute cycle for metal items with lumens and porous items sterilized together with an exposure temperature of 270° F (132° C) [5].

A sterilization log or database should be used. The log should include information on the load, the device process, the patient receiving the item, and the reason for flash sterilization [3]. The log may be developed by the facility or individuals can use the commercially available log sheet developed by the manufacturer of the biological indicators. Carlo [3] provides a sample of a flash sterilization log that can easily be adapted for use in any institution.

Recommendations of the Association for the Advancement of Medical Instrumentation

In 2006, the American National Standards Institute/AAMI (ANSI/AAMI ST79:2006) updated the general concept of sterilization [5] and identified criteria for a flash sterilization cycle:

- The cycle is programmed to a specific time and temperature setting established by the manufacturer, based on the type of sterilizer control, and by the user, based on the type of load.
- The items usually are processed unwrapped. Single wraps may be used only if the manufacturer's instructions permit it. Some rigid container systems are specifically designed and validated by the manufacturer for use with the flash sterilization process.
- The items processed via this cycle are assumed to be wet because of the absence of a drying time.
- Items processed must be used immediately in an aseptic method.
- There is no storage or shelf life for any item processed via flash sterilization.

General procedures to ensure an effective process

Decontamination and preparation are essential components that must be successfully completed when flash sterilization is used. In any method of sterilization, a process practice should be clearly outlined and readily available for the members of the surgical team to review and follow. When performed according to recommended standards, flash sterilization is a safe and effective means to address the issue of emergent sterilization. Guidelines for flash sterilization must stress the need to ensure that cleaning and decontamination occur before processing in a flash sterilizer, and that the processes are designed to protect the health care worker. Also, documentation of the flash sterilization process must be consistent with the practice used in routine processing of wrapped loads. Flash-sterilized instruments must be transported in a safe manner to decrease the possibility of contamination from any other source.

The decision to reprocess instruments by flash sterilization should be considered only if the following conditions are met:

- Work practices ensure proper cleaning and decontamination, inspection and arrangement of instruments into the recommended trays or devices before sterilization.
- The physical layout of the department permits the direct delivery of sterilized items to the point of use.
- Polices and procedures are developed, followed, and monitored to ensure aseptic processes and safety of health care workers during the transfer of the items from the sterilizer to the point of use.
- The item is emergently needed.

The fundamental issues related to all sterilization are driven by the need to monitor the processes and ensure that flash sterilization is only used for emergency situations and not for convenience or inventory control. The continued monitoring and assessment of any process, including the flash sterilization process, will lead to an improvement of that process. The first step in this process is to ensure that the policies and protocols for the practice are in place. The second step is to maintain educational opportunities. The final step is to audit the process [5].

AORN recommends that any item that has been flashed sterilized is recorded and traceable back to a sterilizer and a patient in an event of a biological test failure. This documentation must be a standard practice. In some organizations, computerized record-keeping facilitates the task of monitoring the performance of the staff and the equipment. These policies and procedures should be consistent and standardized throughout the organization. The monitoring of the sterilization process and its documentation must also be standardized with responsibilities clearly defined.

Policies

The review of policies and procedures should be accomplished with an interdisciplinary team. The team may consist of representatives from the operating room staff and management, central sterile processing, infection control, and facilities management (or whoever is responsible for the maintenance of the sterilizers).

Policies and procedures should state the purpose, which is to provide an environment for the patient that will ensure that instruments and supplies in the perioperative setting are free of all viable microorganisms. Policies and procedures must indicate that flash sterilization should only be used in emergency situations. Emergency must be defined. It can reasonably be defined as any circumstance where the patient cannot safely wait for personnel to sterilize the instruments by the conventional wrapped method in a designated autoclave or location, such as in central sterile processing. Another emergency circumstance is when an instrument has been contaminated during a procedure and is needed immediately. Yet another emergency where flash sterilization is justified is when the surgical plan changes intraoperatively.

There should be a protocol that refers to the process of using a flash sterilizer. Remember to include the need to have biological indicators, which are required as quality assurance measures for all sterilization processes. Biological indicators demonstrate that conditions necessary to achieve sterilization were met during the sterilizer cycle being monitored. A biological indicator is a commercially prepared device with a known population of highly resistance spores. The device tests the effectiveness of the method of sterilization being used. Biological indicators are processed daily for flash sterilizers.

Additionally, it may be prudent to include in the policy which individuals will be accountable for implementing and monitoring the flash sterilization process for the area. One such individual would be, for example, the operating room employee responsible for performing flash sterilization. That person needs to ensure that, before items are used, all sterilization parameters are met by checking the sterilizer printout or graph and verifying that the set temperature, pressure, and exposure time are achieved.

Another area in which accountability is critical is in the scheduling process. Prior to the start of the day's schedule there needs to be an assessment of the elective schedule with instrument availability (including implants) and a determination made of whether the procedure can be performed. A determination also needs to be made of whether an implant is required. The patient cannot be placed in the procedural room until the implant is processed and a final negative biological culture result is received. In addition, loaner instrumentation sets must be inventoried for completeness before sterilization. The operator performs daily biological indicator testing on steam sterilizers and completes an instrument set tracking log on all items sterilized and used on each patient.

The operating room management staff are responsible for informing the surgeon of record of any instrumentation or implant issues that result from an unavailable planned instrumentation or implant for the scheduled procedure; for informing central sterile processing of any instrumentation or implant issues that result from unavailable or unsterile surgical instruments; and for completing the sterilization failure report when a positive biological culture is obtained.

Meanwhile, the surgeon of the operative procedure provides information regarding the type of instrumentation set needed (including implants) 96 hours before the elective schedule is printed; provides options for a possible different system or systems to be used when informed that the primary system is unavailable or unsterile and for emergency bookings; and provides a plan and options for instrumentation or implant as per emergency or urgent add-on slip standard.

Central sterile processing is accountable for such items and supplies needed for decontaminating, preparing, and sterilizing surgical instruments for the perioperative services; performs mechanical, chemical, and biological testing of the sterilizers; and maintains records of testing to ensure that the sterilization processes are successful according to the recommendations of relevant manufacturers and regulating agencies. More specifically, central sterile processing:

- Maintains records of all instruments sterilized for a period of 10 years for steam, plasma, and liquid sterilization
- Includes in every surgical instrument pack and internal integrator, a count sheet, an

external chemical indicator and an identifiable label with a barcode

- Provides preoperative services with surgical instrument sets that are free of microorganisms and are safe and ready to use, and performs a biological test on all implants sterilized.

Meanwhile, infection control is responsible for assisting in the validation of the effectiveness of processing procedures. Other roles of infection control are:

- To assist in the development of a quality assurance program and to coordinate and maintain the data on the sterilization failure report
- To be a consultant on sterilization issues and on regulatory issues relating to sterilization
- To be a consultant on the education materials and topics (infection control and sterilization) for staff education

Flash sterilization failures should be detected at any point in the process or just before the use of the medical device. In investigating factors related to a biological failure during flash sterilization, one must look at equipment failure, process failure, human error, procedural errors, and environmental failures. To assist in this investigation, one will need to know the extent of the failure, the cause, and if recalls are necessary [6].

Monitoring tools

In developing a monitoring tool, be certain that a full description of the method is in compliance with the standards of practice. The tool should be shared with the leadership, the central sterile processing department, and the infection control department. The form is used to document the process for identifying the cause of a failed test for sterilization. It should be a one-page tool for use by a health professional to review the reason for failure of the sterilization process and to identify potential problems in the sterilization process. The supervisor in collaboration completes the form with the staff member who performs the testing of the sterilizer. The copy of the form is kept in the departmental files and copies are shared with the team that reviews all biological failures.

Items to include are:

Name of the department where the failure occurred (eg, labor and delivery, main operating room, ambulatory surgery)
Date of report
Date of test collection
Location and number of the sterilizer (If multiple sterilizers are in one area, a method of identification should be in place.)
Corrective actions taken, such as
Machine taken out of service
Instruments recalled; no patient involvement
Instruments recalled; patient involvement (attach list with medical chart number)
Action taken when the department was notified of a failure in the sterilization process
Cause of the reported failure determined by investigation, such as
Failure of validation test after repairs
Machine malfunction
Improper loading trays into machine
Incorrect sterilizer settings
Dirty or clogged filters or drain
Operator procedure error
Corrective action taken so that error doesn't occur again
What, if any, further follow-up is needed
Name of physician notified, if any was notified
Name of contact person from the department

Data

What should be done with the data collected? First, a decision needs to be made on how to analyze the data. Second, a determination is needed to identify what information needs to be monitored. Third, a choice must be made about where the information will be shared. One may wish to call in a quality improvement specialist to assist in the format of the report. One can analyze this information by looking at the number of flash sterilizing processes per 100 cases. The second part of the data examination is to look at the compliance with documentation in the sterilizer logs. Look at the random number of logs over a short period and the percent compliance with the documentation.

Monitoring of compliance to the protocol should be maintained even if flashing is rare. If there appears to be an increase in the use of flashing, an investigation into the cause of the increase is warranted. The reasons for flashing will be documented in the logs maintained for each sterilizer.

In the event there is a need to understand a problem related to flash sterilization, a team should be formed. The team should include members of the surgical services, sterile processing, and infection control. All members of the team should be able to contribute vital information to categorize the "cause of the problem."

The team may be able to categorize potential causes in an orderly manner and to define the problem. Some possible categories include:

- Method, machine, materials, manpower
- Places, procedures, people, policies
- Surroundings, supplies, systems, skills

The identification of a problem usually indicates a systems problem that has occurred on many levels and in multiple departments. During this process, the problem can be identified and steps taken to eliminate it.

The first step for the team is to identify the problem. The objective is to improve the safety, efficacy, and efficiency of the sterilization process as well as the performance of the staff. The team brainstorms the problem and carefully analyzes every stage of the process.

The inclusion in the group of at least one member of all of the departments involved serves as a catalyst for success. Eliminating a problem can "create another problem" if all the essential players are not included because causes that lead to a problem might be left unresolved. A multi-interdisciplinary team will not only help find the problem but will also improve interdisciplinary communication and relationships.

In summary, an increased focus on a culture of safety is essential in health care. When performed according to recommended standards, flash sterilization is a safe and effective means to address the issue of emergent sterilization. Flash sterilization can be effectively and safely accomplished provided that all the steps in the process are rigidly followed.

References

[1] Centers for Disease Control and Prevention, U.S. Department of Health and Human Services. Guidelines for prevention of surgical site infections. 1999 Infect Control Hosp Epidemiol 1999;20(4): 247–78.

[2] Church NB. Surgical service. In: APIC text for infection control and epidemiology. Washington, DC: APIC; 2005. p. 46–5.

[3] Carlo A. The new era of flash sterilization. AORN J 2007;86(1):58–72.

[4] Association of Operating Room Nurses. Recommended practices for sterilization in the perioperative practice settings. Standards, recommended practices and guidelines. Denver (CO): Association of Operating Room Nurses; 2006. p. 631–33.

[5] Association for the Advancement of Medical Instrumentation. ANSI/AMMI ST79:2006—Comprehensive guide to steam sterilization and sterility assurance in health care facilities. Arlington (VA): Association for the Advancement of Medical Instrumentation; 2007.

[6] Clement L, Ames H. Steam sterilization failure investigation: a systematic line of attack. Healthcare Purchasing News, September 2005.

ELSEVIER
SAUNDERS

Perioperative Nursing Clinics 3 (2008) 127–135

PERIOPERATIVE
NURSING
CLINICS

Sterilization and Disinfection in the Operating Room

Kathi Mullaney, BSN, MPH, CIC

Our Lady of Mercy Medical Center, 600 East 233rd Street, Bronx, NY 10466, USA

At some point in our lives, each of us we will be a patient in the health care system. We may even undergo a surgical procedure. Approximately 46.5 million surgical procedures are performed each year in the United States [1]. According to data on procedures monitored by the National Health Safety Network (formerly the National Nosocomial Infection System) from the Centers for Disease Control and Prevention (CDC), 274,098 surgical-site infections occur each year. That's about 2 surgical-site infections per 100 procedures [2].

Experts estimate that each year in the United States as many as 98,000 deaths are caused by or are associated with a hospital-acquired infection (HAI) and an estimated 8205 deaths are associated with surgical-site infections [2]. The numbers are staggering and the impact of medical errors is stunning. The Quality of Health Care in America Project initiated by the Institute of Medicine in June 1998 developed a strategy to improve the quality of health care delivery in the United States by 2010. Eliminating HAIs in hospitals must be a goal for all health care providers. Tremendous resources are directed toward preventing HAIs [3].

A report published by the Pennsylvania Health Care Cost Containment Council identified the actual number of infections reported by 168 hospitals in Pennsylvania in 2005. It revealed that hospitalization was associated with more than 19,000 cases of infections. These infections added nearly 395,000 additional hospital days at a cost approaching $3.5 billion. The average charge for a patient acquiring an infection was $185,000, compared with $31,389 for those who didn't. The infections also increased the length of stay. Patients who contracted infections in the hospital stayed in the hospital five times longer than uninfected patients did. Most sobering was that the mortality rate, which was more than 5.5 times higher among patients who developed HAIs [4]. In addition to the adverse effects to the patients, HAIs lead to increased litigation and class action lawsuits, according to reports from health care facilities. What is most disturbing about these deaths and adverse outcomes is that they are unnecessary and avoidable [5].

Imagine an operating room where an orthopedic surgeon finds that a cannulated drill bit she is using has a guide wire stuck in it from a previous case. Now flecks of hardened, autoclaved blood from another patient have just contaminated her patient's wound.

Imagine also a surgical technician setting up for a procedure and, while preparing instruments on the back table, discovering what looks like blood or tissue in the serrations of a clamp. Before making this discovery, the technician had touched other sterile supplies [6].

Contaminated instruments can cost time, money, and, ultimately, the lives of patients.

Therefore, it is ultimately the responsibility of the perioperative nurse to minimize patient risk for developing a surgical-site infection by implementing instrument-processing recommendations and standards relevant to the operating room. A variety of organizations are involved in formulating these recommendations and standards (Box 1).

In the perioperative setting, patients are subjected to invasive procedures that involve contact with instruments that touch or penetrate patients' sterile tissues or mucous membranes. This equipment must be clean and sterile to decrease the risk of an HAI. To prevent the spread of infectious pathogens to patients, the staff must ensure that the equipment is free from organisms. Following evidence-based practice based on national guidelines, the removal of

---

E-mail address: kmullaney@olmhs.org

Box 1. Organizations involved in instrument-processing recommendations and standards relevant to the operating room

The Association of Perioperative Registered Nurses (AORN)
AORN publishes Recommended Practices on Instruments and Powered Equipment—Care and Cleaning, Sterilization in the Perioperative Practice Setting and Disinfection, High-Level, and Packaging Systems—Selection and Use. These documents are reviewed periodically and updated at least every 5 years.

Association for Advancement of Medical Instrumentation (AAMI)
AAMI is a standards-setting body that includes representatives from the sterilization technology industry, consultants, scientists, and users. The documents published by this organization are frequently referenced by other standards-setting bodies and are considered to be the definitive United States standards for sterilization and disinfection.

International Standards Organization (ISO)
ISO is an international standards-setting body. Many of the ISO sterilization and disinfection standards are adopted in the United States and elsewhere.

The Society for Gastroenterology Nurses and Associates (SGNA)
SGNA writes standards related to reprocessing devices used in gastrointestinal endoscopy.

Association for Professionals in Infection Control and Epidemiology (APIC)
APIC strives to improve health and patient safety by reducing the risk of infection and other adverse outcomes. This is accomplished through education, research, collaboration in the formulation of public policy guidelines, and credentialing.

Society for Healthcare Epidemiology of America (SHEA)
SHEA strives to advance the application of health care epidemiology.

American Society for Gastrointestinal Endoscopy (ASGE)
ASGE is a professional organization dedicated to advancing patient care and digestive health by promoting excellence in endoscopy.

Joint Commission (JC)
Formerly known as the Joint Commission on Accreditation of Healthcare Organizations (JCAHO), JC accredits and certifies health care organizations. It is recognized nationwide as a symbol of quality.

Healthcare Infection Control Practices Advisory Committee (HICPAC)
HICPAC, a division of Healthcare Quality Promotion, is made up of 14 external infection control experts who provide advice and guidance to the CDC and to the Secretary of the Department of Health and Human Services regarding the practice of health care infection control, strategies for surveillance and prevention, and control of health care–associated infections in United States health care facilities.

visible dirt and invisible microorganisms is the most important step in preventing transmission of pathogens to the patient.

Spaulding classification

How a device is used determines how the device must be processed. The Spaulding classification of medical devices, developed by Earle H. Spaulding [7,8] almost 40 years ago, is the standard of practice to disinfect and sterilize patient care items or equipment and is widely accepted by the Food and Drug Administration (FDA), the CDC, epidemiologists, microbiologists and many professional organizations. As outlined in Table 1, the three Spaulding classifications are critical, semicritical, and noncritical.

Critical devices

Critical items come in contact with sterile tissue or the vascular system. Examples of critical devices include scissors, hemostats, and scalpels. These items must be sterilized. Sterilization of these items is achieved through the use of steam, ethylene oxide, hydrogen peroxide gas plasma, or liquid chemical sterilants [1].

Semicritical devices

Semicritical items come in contact with intact mucous membranes or nonintact skin but do not penetrate the skin or other sterile areas of the body. Examples of semicritical items include laryngoscope blades, endoscopes, respiratory therapy equipment, and diaphragm fitting rings. These items may be sterilized and require a minimum of high-level disinfection using chemical disinfectants. High-level disinfection is a process that kills all microorganisms with the exception of a high number of spores. Glutaraldehyde, hydrogen peroxide, ortho-phthaldehyde, peracetic acid with hydrogen peroxide and chlorine are approved by the FDA as high-level disinfectants, provided the parameters of use are met [1].

Noncritical devices

Noncritical items come in contact with intact skin but not mucous membranes. Intact skin provides a natural barrier against microorganisms. Examples of noncritical items include blood pressure cuffs, crutches, stretchers, and linens. These items require low-level disinfection. The use of soap and water represent one example of low-level disinfection [1].

Overview of instrument processing

Cleaning

Cleaning is the most important step in instrument processing. Excellent cleaning practices are essential to advance to the next steps of sterilization. Before the instruments can be used, instrument surfaces must be cleaned. Cleaning is the removal of foreign material (eg, soil or organic material) from objects. This can be accomplished by using water with detergents or enzymatic products. Debris and bioburden must be removed to guarantee the sterilization or disinfection process. Even with a sterilizer working properly, debris remaining on the surfaces of instruments can interfere with the effectiveness of the sterilization and disinfection processes. When the debris becomes dried and baked onto instruments, removal of the debris becomes difficult and the sterilization and disinfection process is compromised.

The cleaning process must be initiated in the operating room by wiping down instruments with a damp cloth and rinsing or soaking the instruments to prevent blood and tissue from drying on the instruments. Following surgery, instruments should be covered and transported to a dedicated decontamination area. Enzyme sprays, gels, and foams can be applied to the surgical instruments to prevent the debris from drying onto instruments awaiting decontamination.

Cleaning can be accomplished manually or mechanically (ultrasonic cleaner or washer-disinfector). Manual cleaning requires friction by vigorous rubbing and scrubbing of the instrument to remove the gross debris. Mechanical cleaning and automated decontamination can also be accomplished in a washer-sterilizer or washer-decontaminator after

Table 1
Classification of medical devices, processes, and products

Spaulding classification	Examples of devices	Process classification	FDA product classification
Critical: enters sterile tissue or vascular system	Scissors, hemostats, scalpels	Sterilization chemical sterilant	Sterilant/disinfection
Semicritical: contact with intact mucous membranes or nonintact skin	Laryngoscope blades, endoscopes, diaphragm rings	High-level disinfectant Pasteurization	Sterilant/disinfection
Noncritical: contact with intact skin	Blood pressure cuffs, stethoscopes, crutches, stretchers, linens	Intermediate, low-level disinfection	Hospital disinfectant with and without tuberculocidal activity

Data from Fauerbach L, Janelle J. Practical applications in infection control. In: Block SS, editor. Disinfection, sterilization and preservation. Philadelphia: Lippincott Williams & Wilkins; 2001. p. 935–44.

the gross debris is removed. The use of an ultrasonic cleaner may be necessary to remove fine debris from crevices or areas difficult to clean. Ultrasonic cleaners use high-frequency sound waves to clean. Scissors and other hinged instruments must be opened to allow adequate contact with the detergent solution. To ensure thorough cleaning, instruments should be disassembled and should not be stacked. Personal protective equipment (impervious gown, utility gloves, and eye protection) should be worn during the cleaning process to prevent exposure to blood and body fluids (Box 2).

Disinfection

Disinfection kills microorganisms on inanimate objects, such as surgical instruments and horizontal surfaces. Disinfection is accomplished by soaking instruments in liquid chemical germicides. Available disinfectants provide either high-, intermediate-, or low-level disinfection. High-level disinfectants kill all vegetative microorganisms (eg, bacteria, mycobacteria, fungi, viruses) and some bacterial spores. They are also tuberculocidal. High-level disinfectants are used on instruments and devices, such as gastroscopes, cystoscopes, and speculums, that come in contact with mucous membranes but do not penetrate the membrane and do not enter sterile body sites. Intermediate-level disinfectants kill most viruses, most fungi, and all vegetative pathogenic bacteria but do not kill spores. Intermediate-level disinfectants are used on floors, walls, and other horizontal surfaces. Low-level disinfectants kill some vegetative bacteria, some fungi, and lipid viruses. They are ineffective against spores and nonlipid viruses and are not tuberculocidal. Low-level disinfectants are used on floors, walls, and other horizontal surfaces [9].

Box 2. Cleaning highlights

- Wear personal protective equipment before starting the cleaning process.
- Cleaning is the most critical step in processing instruments.
- Inadequate cleaning can compromise the sterilization process.
- Cleaning can be accomplished without sterilizing; sterilizing cannot be accomplished without cleaning.

Examples of disinfectants include:

- High-level disinfectants: aldehydes (eg, glutaraldehyde, ortho-phthalaldehyde), hydrogen peroxide, and peracetic acid
- Intermediate-level disinfectants: sodium hypochlorite and isopropyl alcohol
- Low-level disinfectants: quaternary ammonium compounds, hydrogen peroxide, and phenols [10]

Check manufacturers' guidelines when selecting disinfectants. When using a disinfectant, follow the manufacturer's recommendations for concentration, temperature, and contact time. The manufacturer's instructions should be followed when preparing the disinfectant solution and calculating the expiration dates. Some disinfectants can be used for different levels of disinfection or even for sterilization, depending on their exposure time or concentration. The most common high-level disinfectants include glutaraldehyde and ortho-phthalaldehyde.

Glutaraldehyde

Exposing a clean, dry instrument to a 2.5% glutaraldehyde solution for 20 minutes at room temperature provides high-level disinfection. Exposure for 10 hours at 77°C results in sterilization. Instruments intended for high-level disinfection must be cleaned thoroughly and dried before disinfection. Moisture on instruments can dilute the disinfectant solution. Test strips specific to the chemical agent and the minimum effective concentration of the chemical must be used to monitor the effectiveness of the solution [11].

Ortho-phthalaldehyde

Exposing a clean, dry instrument to a 0.55% ortho-phthalaldehyde solution for 12 minutes at room temperature results in high-level disinfection. There is no mixing or activation. The solution has a maximum life of 14 days. The solution has little odor, which decreases irritability to the user [11].

Safety precautions

Disinfectant safety precautions include (Box 3):

- Wearing appropriate personal protective equipment to protect mucous membranes.
- Mixing and using glutaraldehyde solutions in a well-ventilated designated area or a room with a minimum of 10 air exchanges.

- Storing the solutions in a closed, covered container.
- In-servicing staff yearly on the safe use of the solutions.
- Implementing a spill procedure.
- Providing an eyewash station near the point of use.

Sterilization

Sterilization is the complete elimination or destruction of all forms of microbial life. It is measured by the probability of viable microorganisms being present on a device after sterilization. This probability is referred to as a sterility assurance level (SAL) and is expressed in mathematical terms. The standard in the health care industry is 10^{-6}. This mathematical expression means there is no more than one in a million chance that any viable microorganisms can remain on a device after sterilization. Manufacturers of sterilizing equipment must demonstrate the SAL to the FDA before the technology can be used to sterilize medical devices. Methods of sterilization include the use of steam, ethylene oxide, peracetic acid, dry heat, and hydrogen peroxide gas plasma. No matter how technologically advanced the sterilization process, sterilization can only occur if the device is clean, inspected, and packaged before the sterilization process. Medical devices that contact sterile body tissues or fluids are considered critical items. Critical items must be sterile to prevent the risk of infection [1].

Box 3. Disinfection highlights

- Wear personal protective equipment during the disinfection process.
- Disinfectants are used only on inanimate objects.
- Disinfectant solutions of 2% to 3.2% glutaraldehyde and 0.55% ortho-phthalaldehyde are the most common high-level disinfectants used in the operating room.
- Instruments should be dry before being submerged in solution to avoid diluting the disinfectant solution.
- When using disinfectant solutions, follow manufacturer's recommendations for concentration, temperature, and contact time.

Preparation

Before the sterilization process, instruments must be:

1. Soaked in an enzymatic detergent promptly after use to remove all debris
2. Disassembled
3. Cleaned according to the manufacturer's recommendations and including lumen, serrations, teeth, jaws, and hinges
4. Thoroughly rinsed and the lumen flushed with water
5. Inspected after the cleaning process for cleanliness, proper function and alignment, defects, sharpness, and chipping of plated surfaces.
6. Secured in the open position if handled instruments
7. Allowed to thoroughly dry
8. Placed in trays designated for the sterilization process [12]

Packaging

Medical devices should be packaged so that sterility is achieved and maintained to the point of use. Packaging products include wraps (textile or nonwoven), peel pouches, and containers (metal or plastic). Packaging must allow penetration of the sterilant, remain durable inside and outside the sterilizer, repel moisture and water, and be made of material with low-lint characteristics. Proper packaging techniques must be implemented to ensure sterilization of the instruments. Correctness in order of the instruments, direction of folds, and the number of wraps is important to maintain sterility, reduce contamination, and keep items clean, dry, and intact until use. The surgical packs and pouches should have labels that state their contents and the date of sterilization. Sterility is event-related, not time-related. Instruments packaged correctly, handled minimally, rotated so the oldest package is used first, and stored in a clean, dry, cool, and contained environment are considered sterile unless the package is damaged [13].

Sterilization processing choices

The choice of sterilization process depends on the ability of the instrument to withstand heat. Sterilization processes include steam sterilization (using autoclaves), ethylene oxide sterilization, gas plasma sterilization, and peracetic acid sterilization.

Steam sterilization is the most common, reliable, and economical sterilization process for heat- and moisture-stable instruments. Moisture is added to accelerate the process of microbial destruction. Pressure above atmospheric pressure is necessary to increase the temperature of the steam for thermal destruction of microbial life. The basis of the steam sterilization process is direct saturated steam contact. For a required time and at a specified temperature, the steam must penetrate every fiber and reach every surface of the items being sterilized. The packages should be packed loosely to allow free movement of steam and prevent entrapment of air and water. The three critical parameters— time, temperature, and steam saturation—must be met for the steam sterilization process to be achieved [11]. Table 2 provides information on the different types of sterilizers and the parameters required to achieve sterilization.

Flash sterilization, steam sterilization of an unwrapped instrument, takes much less time than sterilization of a wrapped instrument. Flash sterilization should only be used for items that are needed immediately and for which there is no immediate replacement. Flash sterilization should not be used for implantable devices [14]. Table 3 provides information on types of flash sterilizers and the required parameters for each. When using the flash sterilization process, the following guidelines must be followed:

- Instruments must be properly cleaned, decontaminated, inspected, and placed in the appropriate container before sterilization.

Table 2
Steam sterilization parameters for loads with porous and nonporous items

Type of sterilizer	Time	Temperature
Gravity displacement	15–30 min	250°–254°F (121°–123°C)
	10–25 min	270°–272°F (132°–135°C)
Prevacuum	3–4 min	270°–272°F (132°–135°C)
Steam-flush/pressure pulse	20 min	250°–254°F (121°–123°C)
	3–4 min	270°–272°F (132°–135°C)

From Fogg DM. Infection prevention and control. In: Meeker MH, Rothrock JC, editors. Alexander's care of the patient in surgery. Philadelphia: WB Saunders; 1999. p. 97–158; with permission.

- The sterilization process must be completed close to point of use.
- Precautions must be taken to ensure the item can be delivered sterile and safely to the point of use.
- Documentation must be maintained of flashed items for each cycle.

The Association of periOperative Registered Nurses (AORN) Recommended Practice for Sterilization in Perioperative Practice Settings states:

Flash sterilization should only be used in carefully selected clinical situations when certain parameters are met. Flash sterilization should only be used when there is insufficient time to process by the preferred wrapped or container method. Flash sterilization should not be used as a substitute for sufficient instrument inventory [15].

CDC guidelines state that "flash sterilization is not intended to be used for either reasons of convenience or as an alternative to purchasing more instruments or to save time" [16].

Ethylene oxide sterilization is used for temperature-sensitive devices, such as cameras, endoscopes, and electrical cables. The critical parameters for ethylene oxide are gas concentration, temperature, humidity, and exposure time. Ethylene oxide is classified as a known carcinogen, is highly flammable, and requires hours for sterilization and aeration. Ethylene oxide sterilizers operate at low temperatures and humidity, typically between 130°F to 140°F (49°C–60°C) and 40% to 60% humidity for 2.5 hours of sterilization time, with 12 to 18 hours of aeration time. The required exposure time depends on temperature, humidity, gas concentration, ease of penetration, and type of organism to be destroyed. The Occupational Safety and Health Administration has issued standards regulating employee exposure to ethylene oxide and requires close monitoring of employees. Perioperative nurses in the operating room are rarely responsible for ethylene oxide sterilization. However, nurses could be exposed to potential harm if the lengthy cycles required for ethylene oxide sterilization are cut short [17].

Because ethylene oxide sterilization is time consuming, costly, and a potential hazard to the staff, alternatives have been sought. New sterilization technologies that have emerged include hydrogen peroxide gas plasma, which is suitable for heat-sensitive items, and peracetic acid,

Table 3
Flash steam sterilization parameters

Type of sterilizer	Load configuration	Time	Temperature
Gravity displacement	Metal/nonporous (no lumen)	3 min	270°–272°F (132°–135°C)
	Metal with lumen and porous	10 min	270°–272°F (132°–135°C)
Prevacuum	Metal/nonporous (no lumen)	3 min	270°–272°F (132°–135°C)
	Metal with lumen and porous	4 min (or manufacturer's recommendations)	270°–272°F (132°–135°C)
Pulsing gravity	Nonporous, nonlumened	Follow manufacturer's instructions	
Abbreviated prevacuum	Nonporous, nonlumened	Follow manufacturer's instructions	

From Fogg DM. Infection prevention and control. In: Meeker MH, Rothrock JC, editors. Alexander's care of the patient in surgery. Philadelphia: WB Saunders; 1999. p. 97–158; with permission.

a point-of-use technology commonly used to sterilize endoscopes.

Managing contaminated items with prion disease

Prions are resistant to routine disinfection and sterilization methods. Thus, special procedures are needed for transmissible spongiform encephalopathy and Creutzfeldt-Jakob disease. Recommendations on how to manage and reprocess prion-contaminated items can be found in World Health Organization, CDC and AORN publications. In general, it involves sterilization for a longer period of time—approximately 18 minutes to 60 minutes—and at higher temperatures—ranging from 121°C to 132°C, depending on whether the autoclave is a prevacuum or gravity-displacement model [1].

Sterilization process quality-control measures

The sterilization process must be tested on a regular basis to ensure that all parameters of sterilization are met, that the equipment is functioning properly, and that the sterilization process is effective. Monitors are available in three types: mechanical, chemical, and biological.

Mechanical monitors

Mechanical monitors measure the duration of exposure to the sterilant and are built into the sterilizer. The parameters that must be monitored for steam sterilization include time, temperature, and pressure. Steam sterilizers provide a printout that documents the temperature, the pressure, and the length of steam exposure. The data on the printout should be considered only as a measure of effectiveness in sterilizing a particular package. Effectiveness must be measured with chemical or biological indicators. The sterilizer provides a printout for each load. That printout should be filed for future reference. Mechanical monitors are externally attached to the sterilizer, can be read by the staff, and provide real-time quality measurements.

Chemical indicators

Chemical indicators detect sterilization failures that may be a result of incorrect packaging, incorrect loading, or sterilizer malfunction. There are five classes of chemical indicators. Always check the indicator before placing the items on the sterile field.

Class I indicator. A class I indicator determines whether an item has been processed. This type of indicator can be tape, a strip of paper, or a label that changes color during the sterilization process. It only indicates the sterilization process occurred. It does not indicate the items were sterilized.

Class II indicator. A class II indicator, also known as a Bowie-Dick indicator, tests the ability of the high or prevacuum steam sterilizer's ability to create a vacuum.

Class III indicator. A class III indicator is a single-parameter indicator that reacts to one of the critical parameters of sterilization, such as temperature. The indicator is placed in the center of the packaged items. After the sterilization process is complete, the indicator reveals whether the center of the pack was exposed to a specific temperature. The single-parameter indicator does not indicate whether or not the contents of the package were sterilized.

Class IV indicator. A class IV indicator is a multiple-parameter indicator that reacts to all the critical parameters of sterilization by changing color or showing a wicking change from a pass to fail range. The indicator is placed inside the center of the packaged item.

Class V indicator. A class V indicator is an integrating indicator placed in the center of the packaged items. It reacts to all critical parameters of sterilization. The integrator verifies that all conditions for sterilization are met and that the packaged items are sterile [18]. Class V indicators provides a higher level of sterility assurance than class I, III, or IV indicators.

Biological indicators

Biological indicators challenge the sterilization cycle. The biological indicators test the sterilizer's ability to kill highly resistant organisms. A biological indicator can be an ampoule, strip, or capsule impregnated with either *Geobacillus stearothermophilus* for steam, hydrogen peroxide, and peracetic acid processors, or *Bacillus atrophaeus* for ethylene oxide processors. The biological indicator is placed in a test pack, processed in the sterilizer, and then placed in an incubator for at least 24 hours. No growth indicates a negative result, which means the sterilizer is functioning effectively. AORN recommends daily monitoring of steam sterilizers and peracetic acid processors, especially when sterilizing loads contain steam-sterilized implants, but at least weekly. AORN recommends daily monitoring of ethylene oxide sterilizers and following the manufacturers recommendations for hydrogen peroxide gas plasma equipment. If the biological indicator is positive, do not release the load and recall released loads. Investigate the cause of the positive result. Implement an ongoing preventative maintenance schedule for all sterilizers [18].

Future guidelines

Updated Guidelines on Facility Disinfection and Sterilization is anticipated to be released from the Healthcare Infection Control Practices Advisory Committee in the near future. The last related document, Guidelines for Handwashing and Hospital Environmental Control, was published in 1985 and included a section on cleaning, disinfecting, and sterilizing equipment.

Surgical conscience

Develop your "surgical conscience" by improving your knowledge of aseptic technique, developing your self-awareness related to your chosen profession, making intelligent practice decisions, and gathering the courage to make decisions that eliminate the patient's risk of developing an HAI [19]. Implement rigorous standards that include enforcing a strict hand hygiene program, meticulous cleaning of equipment and the environment between patients, requiring strict aseptic technique, and improving communication among all staff members. Above all, maintain a high level of knowledge related to cleaning, disinfection, and sterilization. These critical steps can ensure excellent infection prevention best practices for your surgical patients.

References

[1] Rutala WA, Weber DJ. An overview of disinfection and sterilization in healthcare facilities. In: Rutala WA, editor. Disinfection, sterilization and antisepsis. Principles, practices, current issues and new research. Washington, DC: Association for Professionals in Infection Control and Epidemiology, Inc.; 2006. p. 12–36, 17, 18, 20, 31.

[2] Klevens RM, Edwards JR, Richards CL, et al. Estimating health-care associated infections and deaths in U.S. hospitals, 2002. Public Health Rep 2007; 122:160–5.

[3] Klevens RM, Edwards JR, Richards CL, et al. A comprehensive approach to improving patient safety. In: Kohn LT, Corrigan Janet, Donaldson Molla S, editors. To err is human: building a safer health system. Washington, DC: National Academy Press; 2000. p. 17–25.

[4] Pennsylvania Healthcare Cost Containment Council. Research brief: hospital-acquired infections in Pennsylvania 2005. PHC4. 2005.

[5] Maxfield D. Silence kills. Managing Infection Control 2006;5:32–7.

[6] Johnson S. Decontamination and sterilization: When it comes to reprocessing you can't have one or the other. Outpatient Magazine 2006;5:10–8.

[7] Favero MS, Bond WW. Chemical disinfection of medical and surgical materials. In: Block SS, editor. Disinfection, sterilization and preservation. Philadelphia: Lippincott Williams & Wilkins; 2001. p. 881–917.

[8] Fauerbach L, Janelle J. Practical applications in infection control. In: Block SS, editor. Disinfection, sterilization and preservation. Philadelphia: Lippincott Williams & Wilkins; 2001. p. 935–44.

[9] Association of periOperative Registered Nurses. Recommended practices for high-level disinfection. AORN J 2005;81:402–12.

[10] Rutala WA. APIC guidelines for selection and use of disinfectants. Am J Infect Control 1996;24: 313–42.

[11] Advanced Sterilization Products. Aseptic technique in the operating room. Available at: https://www. sterrad.com/Professional_Education. Accessed July, 2007.

[12] Caveney L. Cleaning, disinfection and sterilization. Veterinary Technician 2006;27(4):236–42.

[13] Vyhlidal SK. Central services. In: APIC text of infection control and epidemiology. Washington, DC: Association for Professional in Infection Control and Epidemiology, Inc.; 2005. p. 56–1/56–16.

[14] Association for the Advancement of Medical Instrumentation. Flash sterilization: steam sterilization of patient care items for immediate use. Arlington (VA): AAMI; 2006.

[15] Association of peri-Operative Registered Nurses. Recommended practices for sterilization in the perioperative practice setting. AORN J 2002;75:510–25.

[16] Mangram AJ, Horan TC, Pearson ML, et al. Guidelines for prevention of surgical site infection. Centers for Disease Control and Prevention (CDC) Hospital Infection Control Practices Advisory Committee. Am J Infect Control 1999;27:97–132.

[17] Association for the Advancement of Medical Instrumentation. Ethylene oxide sterilization in health care facilities: safety and effectiveness. Arlington (VA): AAMI; 2006.

[18] Association for the Advancement of Medical Instrumentation. Quality control. Arlington (VA): AAMI; 2006.

[19] Girard NJ. Surgical conscience: still pertinent. AORN J 2007;86(1):13–4.

ELSEVIER
SAUNDERS

Perioperative Nursing Clinics 3 (2008) 137–142

PERIOPERATIVE
NURSING
CLINICS

Infection Prevention for Construction and Renovation in the Operating Room

Sandra Hardy, RN, MA*, Janet P. Haas, RN, DNSc

Infection Prevention and Control Department, New York University Medical Center, New York, NY, USA

Surgical procedures, a necessary part of medical treatment, are intended to improve function and quality of life for patients. However, surgery places patients at risk for complications, including infections. Risk factors for infection include the environment, in addition to the procedure itself and the health care workers in the room. Several reports of infections following surgery have implicated construction in or near the operating room (OR) suite [1–4]. The most frequently reported infections involve cardiac, ophthalmology, and dental surgeries.

The organisms that most frequently cause construction-related infections are *Aspergillus fumigatus* and *Aspergillus flavus* [5,6]. *Aspergillus* is a species of fungus that is ubiquitous in soil, decaying vegetation, household dust, and building material. *Aspergillus* is transmitted by small spores that become suspended in the air and can survive for prolonged periods. Transmission during surgery is by contact of aspergillus spores with the moist tissues of the surgical site. The epidemiology of aspergillus infections related to the OR differs from the usual presentation, in which inhalation of spores leads to invasive infections of both the upper and lower respiratory tracts in a susceptible (usually immune-compromised) host. Invasive aspergillus disease causes high morbidity and even mortality. Ensuring that construction sites in and near ORs are controlled is the best prevention for this devastating complication of surgery.

During construction, as floors, walls, and ceilings are penetrated, or soil is disturbed, spores are liberated and travel in dust or dirt particles. Chances of inhalation or environmental contamination increase. Tabbara and Jabarti [3] reported an outbreak of aspergillus endophthalmitis after cataract extraction during hospital construction. Five patients developed postoperative eye infections. In all five cases, cultures of aqueous or vitreous grew *A fumigatus*. All fives cases occurred in a 3-week period coinciding with hospital construction. Overberger and colleagues [7] showed the effectiveness of preventive measures in decreasing the risk of aspergillus infections during construction. In this study, the construction zone was placed under negative pressure and separated by erection of temporary barriers. Once all measures were in place, air samples from various locations both inside and outside the construction zone before, during, and after a 30-week construction project were taken. In the construction zone, total particulate concentrations and spore counts were elevated, while outside the barriers they did not change significantly from baseline levels.

The American Institute of Architects (AIA) publishes guidelines for hospital design and construction. These have become the basis by which compliance is measured [8,9]. Regulators, such as the Joint Commission, the federal government, and some states, require hospitals and other health care facilities to design, construct, and renovate according to AIA guidelines. Construction projects can be divided into the preconstruction, construction, and postconstruction periods. Each has specific tasks that must be completed to ensure safety of patients in the area.

---

* Corresponding author.
E-mail address: sandra.hardy@nyumc.org
(S. Hardy).

1556-7931/08/$ - see front matter © 2008 Elsevier Inc. All rights reserved.
doi:10.1016/j.cpen.2008.01.004

Preconstruction

The first part of the preconstruction phase is the design phase. AIA guidelines state: "Design and planning for such [renovation and new construction] projects shall require consultation from infection control and safety personnel." Early involvement in the conceptual phase helps ascertain the risks to susceptible patients and disruption of essential patient services [10]. The involvement of the infection control professional (IPC) helps ensure that space and equipment essential to infection prevention is not overlooked in the design. Some of these items include ample storage space for clean supplies, soiled utility rooms, and hand washing facilities. The IPC should be versed in the AIA requirements for the OR or procedure rooms because there are specific requirements for air flow, temperature, and humidity in these areas. The IPC doesn't act alone, but rather becomes a part of a multidisciplinary team that includes architectural and engineering designers, the OR nursing director and nurse manager, surgeons, the facilities department, safety or environmental services, and the hospital or health care administrator [10–12]. Others can be added to the team as appropriate for the organization and the project in question. Each member of this team brings expertise in a particular area. Together the group can best decide how the OR space will function as a whole.

An essential part of the preconstruction phase is developing the Infection Control Risk Assessment (ICRA). The ICRA takes into consideration the type of construction or renovation being done, the amount of time the project will take, and the area of the facility in which the project will be done. The Association for Professionals in Infection Control and Epidemiology has developed a guide to the types of infection control precautions needed based on these factors [12–14]. Appendix 1 shows the version of the construction guideline matrix at the authors' hospital. The focus of infection control during construction is on containing dust and moisture. It is important to document what types of barriers will be needed, what protection is required for elevators that will be used, and what type of cleanup is required. In addition, the ICRA should delineate the routes that construction workers will take getting to and from the project site, the protective clothing or actions required (such as requirements that workers vacuum themselves with a high-efficiency particulate air [HEPA] filter vacuum system to remove dust), and the routes for materials and debris. Depending upon the project, the ICRA may be completed during a preconstruction walk-through before the project begins. However, for larger projects, the AIA now requires preconstruction drawings to include barrier locations and descriptions of how they are to be built [10,11]. It may not be possible to actually walk through the spaces in these cases, so the ICRA is then based on drawings of the project. It is important to have all infection-prevention and environmental-safety measures documented before the project is sent out for bid because these measures will add costs that should be estimated by contractors. Clearly documenting the requirements also gives all parties something to refer to as the project progresses.

A construction and renovation policy (CRP) ensures that management understands the ICRA and specifies essential participants [10]. Following the CRP ensures a safe environment for patients, visitors, and employees during construction projects or repairs of the facility; and provides guidance for project managers, engineers, environmental service workers, and department heads. It determines who has the authority to stop the project and for what reasons, as well as who has authority to restart the project. It includes expectations for contractor accountability in the event of breaches in infection control practices and related agreements [10].

Before construction or renovation in the OR, all construction personnel should be educated about the potential risks to patients and the rationale and strategies for infection prevention during the project. The education includes information regarding the pathogen *Aspergillus* and its transmission, the type of barriers used to contain the dust, and airflow considerations for maintaining negative pressure in the construction area, even though the OR is under positive pressure [9,10,14].

In addition, construction workers must be informed of the routes they should use to enter and exit the construction area, and how to get needed tools and material to the site. To promote understanding, educational material should be provided in the language of the workers if at all possible. To ensure that time is set aside for this important education, the construction contact should require subcontractors and workers to attend [10–12]. OR staff must also be educated about the importance of infection prevention during construction, and told to contact the appropriate OR manager, or even the construction project manager, if barriers are not intact or if work practices are unsafe.

Construction

Infections have been transmitted through the dissemination of microorganisms from disruption of environmental reservoirs (eg, drywall, ceiling tiles, flooring casework) [5]. Before beginning construction, patient supplies and equipment should be removed from the construction site. Any equipment that cannot be moved should be sealed tightly in plastic. Barriers must be erected around virtually all construction or renovation sites in the OR. The specific type of physical barrier required depends on the project's scope, duration, degree of activity (generation of high or low levels of dust), and local fire codes. The OR is considered one of the highest risk areas because of the invasive nature of surgical procedures and the underlying health issues of the population served [9,10]. For short-term projects, such as installation of new cables in the semirestricted area, a portable plastic enclosure from ceiling height to floor with flaps that overlap by at least 2 ft for entry access may be sufficient. For larger and longer term projects, the barrier may include a plastic dust abatement curtain before construction of the rigid barrier; sealing and taping all joint edges, including the top and bottom; extending the barrier from floor to ceiling; and fitting or sealing any temporary doors connecting the construction zone to the adjacent area. An entry vestibule for changing clothes and storing tools is needed for larger jobs. Many facilities are now posting the ICRA at the entrance to the construction site. This communicates compliance with the ICRA requirement, and displays the requirements for barriers and other infection prevention measures openly for all to follow.

Special ventilation is required during construction. Under normal conditions, ORs are maintained under positive pressure with air introduced at the ceiling and exhausted near the floor [15]. This means that air flows from the operating room toward the corridors and adjacent areas. During construction, the air within the construction area must be contained [9,10,14]. Fans should be turned off before opening ductwork. Adjacent areas should be evaluated to ensure there are no hidden wall or ceiling penetrations [9,10]. One of the first steps in preparing for construction is to isolate the ventilation system in the area. Air exhaust from the construction site should be directed outside via a window with no recirculation into the building.

If the exhaust must tie into a recirculation air system, a prefilter and HEPA filter unit are used before exhaust to prevent contamination of the ducts. In addition, the construction site must be under negative pressure with respect to surrounding areas. The construction personnel or the facilities department must maintain and monitor the negative pressure. This can be done with a smoke test similar to that used for tuberculosis isolation rooms, or with mechanical monitors. The results should be documented, and some facilities choose to post the results of monitoring at the entrance to the construction site as well as keeping them on file.

During construction and renovation, specific traffic patterns should be established and maintained. Designated entry and exit procedures should have been defined in the preconstruction phase [9,10,12]. While construction is occurring, operating room personnel must be able to move from place to place without contaminating their surgical scrubs. Clean or sterile supplies and equipment must be transported to storage areas by a route that minimizes the potential for contamination from any source [10,14]. During construction, this includes construction materials and debris along with the usual OR soiled or contaminated trash and linen. Hallways, elevators, entrances, and exits for construction workers must be designated and clearly marked [10,12]. Patients may not be transported on the same elevator with construction material and debris.

If traffic patterns are not easily altered to meet these requirements, then construction personnel may need to work during off-hours or weekends. If infection control requirements still cannot be met, the area may need to be relocated or closed temporarily [10]. Any decision to relocate or temporarily close should be made by the multidisciplinary planning team. The ICRA incorporates a list of guidelines for movement of supplies, equipment, and debris.

Construction workers entering the semirestricted and restricted area should be provided with disposable jump suits, head and shoe covers. Protective clothing should be removed before exiting the work area. Tools and equipment should be damp-wiped before being transported from the work area. In unrestricted areas, protective apparel is not always worn. In cases where workers don't wear protective clothing, an HEPA-filtered vacuum should be used to remove dust from clothing before leaving the construction site [8,9,12]. The construction area should be maintained in a clean manner by contractors and swept

Appendix 1

Construction matrix used at New York University medical center

Construction Matrix used at NYU Medical Center

CONSTRUCTION PRECAUTIONS NEEDED TO PREVENT INFECTIONS IN PATIENTS

INSTRUCTIONS: Locate the type of work that is planned (Type A, B, C, or D) along the top row of the grid, then find the area of planned construction in left column (Group 1, 2, 3, or 4). The intersecting area in the grid tells the class of work (CLASS I, II, III or IV) and the precautions that are needed.

Construction activity CLASS grid (By area and type of work)	Type A Inspection and noninvasive activities. Includes, but is not limited to, removal of ceiling tiles for visual inspection limited to 1 tile per 50 square feet, painting (but no sanding), wall-covering, electrical trim work, minor plumbing and activities which do not generate dust or require cutting of walls or access to ceilings other than for visual inspection.	Type B Small scale, short duration activities which create minimal dust. Includes, but is not limited to, installation of phone and computer cabling, access to chase spaces, cutting of walls or ceilings where dust migration can be controlled.	Type C Any work which generates a moderate to high level of dust or requires demolition or removal of any fixed building components or assemblies. Includes, but is not limited to, sanding of walls for painting or wall covering, removal of floor coverings, ceiling tiles or casework, new wall construction, minor duct work or electrical work above ceilings, major cabling activities and any work that can not be completed in one shift.	Type D Major demolition and construction projects. Includes, but is not limited to, activities which require consecutive shifts, heavy demolition or removal of a complete cabling system and new construction.
Group 1 Office areas Non patient care areas not otherwise specified.(NOS)	**CLASS I** 1. Execute work by methods to minimize raising dust. 2. Immediately replace any ceiling tiles displaced for visual inspection.	**CLASS II (All of precautions for CLASS I, plus)** 1. Isolate area with barriers or provide active means to prevent airborne dust from dispersing into atmosphere. 2. Seal unused doors with masking tape. 3. Block off and seal air vents 4. Wipe surfaces with disinfectant. 5. Provide adhesive walk off mats at entrance and exit of work area.	**CLASS III**	**CLASS III** (See instructions for Class III)
Group 2 Cardiology/Echocardiology Endoscopy/Nuclear Medicine/MRI Radiology/PhysicalTherapy/ Respiratory Therapy	**CLASS II** (See instructions for class II)		**CLASS III**	**CLASS IV (All of precautions for CLASS I, II & III, plus)** 1. Seal holes, pipes, conduits and punctures appropriately. 2. Create an anteroom if necessary. 3. DO NOT remove barriers from work area until completed project thoroughly cleaned by the Building Services Dept and is inspected by Environmental Services and Infection Surveillance Departments.
Group 3 CCU/ Emergency Department/Labor and Delivery/Laboratories/Newborn Nursery/ Outpatient surgery/Pediatrics/Pharmacy/PACU Surgical Units	**CLASS II** (See instructions for class II)	**CLASS III**		
Group 4 Cardiac Cath lab (?) Central Sterile Supply/IntensiveCare Units/Medical Units/Oncology Unit/ Operating Rooms (including C-section rooms in L.&D)	**CLASS II** (See instructions for class II)	**CLASS III (All of precautions for CLASS I & II, plus)** 1. Project mgr. to notify Infection Surveillance and Environmental Services Depts before construction begins. 2. Isolate HVAC system where work is being done to prevent contamination of duct system. 3. Complete all barriers before construction begins, or use Control Cube Method. 4. Post signs as necessary. 5. Use plastic barriers above ceiling tiles. 6. Maintain negative air pressure within the work site or use HEPA filtration units, when necessary. 7. Wear paper coveralls and shoe coverings for wall demolition or other activities creating excessive dust, Remove each time workers leave the work site. 8. Use moist direct route to the outside for waste removal and contain construction waste in tightly covered containers before transport. 9. Cover transport carts and tape covering. 10. Remove barriers carefully to minimize spread of dirt and construction debris. 11. Wet mop and/or Vacuum with HEPA filtered vacuum before leaving work area.		

or HEPA-vacuumed daily or more frequently as needed. Walk-off mats help minimize tracking of heavy dirt and dust from the construction area [9,10]. The construction site must be frequently monitored to ensure compliance with the ICRA [10,12] and maintenance of appropriate air-pressure relationships [9,10]. The use of a checklist provides a way to ensure that all aspects of the site are monitored daily. The project manager or designee is usually responsible for day-to-day monitoring of the construction site, with the ICP also checking the area often. Some facilities have a designated person who monitors construction sites and oversees the infection control and safety aspects of construction projects.

Throughout the construction or renovation project, the facilities or maintenance department should monitor and evaluate the air-pressure differentials and humidity within the construction zone (negative pressure) and the adjacent OR (positive pressure) to ensure that the ventilation system is functioning properly. Any concerns identified should be brought to the attention of the ICP and project manager or, if required, to the multidisciplinary team.

Postconstruction

Before the construction area can be returned to full service or patient occupancy, the multidisciplinary team should walk through and inspect the area. A tool that has been used by contractors is a "punch list," which ensures missed details have been addressed (eg, hand washing sinks, installation of soap) [10].

A cleanup agreement is established in the early planning phase. This agreement delineates who is responsible for the various aspects of cleanup and final cleaning after removal of barriers. The facilities department restores appropriate air condition and heating equipment, and cleans or replaces filters [9,10]. Before the OR suite can be occupied, an environmental air sampling is conducted to evaluate for potential sources of airborne fungal spores that can be detrimental to a patient undergoing surgery [5,9–11]. States and localities may require inspection before the OR can be open for use. Check your state or city regulations.

Summary

Construction and renovation projects in the operating room can increase the risk of invasive aspergillus infections among patients having surgery during these activities. A proactive approach minimizes the risk of infections. A multidisciplinary team is required to plan and implement preventive measures throughout the construction project. The OR staff and leadership play an important role in the planning of new or renovated facilities and especially in monitoring the construction site within their work area. Appropriate preventive measures during OR construction help to promote patient safety.

References

[1] Pasqualotto AC, Denning DW. Post-operative aspergillosis. Clin Microbiol Infect 2006;12:1060–76.

[2] Diaz-Guerra TM, Mellado E, Cuenca-Estrella M, et al. Genetic similarity among one aspergillus flavus strain isolated from a patient who underwent heart surgery and two environmental strains obtained from the operating room. J Clin Microbiol 2000; 38:2419–22.

[3] Tabbara KF, Jabarti AA. Hospital construction–associated outbreak of ocular aspergillosis after cataract surgery. Ophthalmology 1998;105:522–6.

[4] Sanchez RO, Hernandez JM. Infection control during construction and renovation in the operating room. Semin Perioper Nurs 1999;8(4):208–14.

[5] Cooper EE, O'Reilly MA, Guestand DI, et al. Influence of building construction work on Aspergillus infection in a hospital setting. Infect Control Hosp Epidemiol 2003;24:472–6.

[6] Vonberg R-P, Gatmeier P. Noscomial aspergillosis in outbreak settings. J Hosp Infect 2006;63:246–54.

[7] Overberger PA, Wadowsky RM, Schaper MM. Evaluation of airborne particulates and fungi during hospital renovation. Am Ind Hyg Assoc J 1995;56: 706–12.

[8] The American Institute of Architects and Facilities Guidelines Institute. Guidelines for design and construction of hospitals and health care facilities. Washington (DC): American Institute of Architects Press 2001. 5.1 A; p. 15.

[9] Centers for Disease Control and Prevention. Guidelines for environmental infection control in health care facilities. MMWR 2003;53(RR10):1–42.

[10] Bartley JM, the 1997, 1998 and 1999 APIC Guidelines Committee. APIC state-of-art report: the role of infection control during construction in healthcare facilities. Am J Infect Control 2000;28:156–69.

[11] Hansen W. Infection control during construction. Manual; policies, procedures, and strategies for compliance. 2nd. Marblehead (MA): HCPro, Inc. 2004. p. 24–41, 185, 214–19.

[12] Health Canada. Construction-related nosocominal infection in patients in health care facilities: decreasing the risk of aspergillus, legionella and other infections. Can Commun Dis Rep 2001;27(Suppl 2):1–46.

[13] Streifel AJ, Hendrickson C. Assessment of health risks related to construction. HPAC Heating/Piping/AirConditioning Engineering 2002;27–32.

[14] Association of Operating Room Nurse. Standards, recommended practices guidelines. Denver (CO): Association of Operating Room Nurses 2006.

[15] Streifel AJ. Health-care IAQ guidance for infection control. HPAC Heating/Piping/AirConditioning Engineering 2000;28–36.

ELSEVIER
SAUNDERS

Perioperative Nursing Clinics 3 (2008) 143–148

PERIOPERATIVE
NURSING
CLINICS

Operating Room Sanitation: Routine Cleaning Versus Terminal Cleaning

Mary Ann Magerl, RN, MA, CIC

Infection Control Department, Westchester Medical Center, 18 Massachusetts Drive,
Valhalla, New York 12550, USA

In the past, surgical procedures were conducted in an operation theater. Today, most surgeries take place in operating rooms (ORs). The theaters were auditorium-type rooms with raised surgical tables over a central stage. The surgery being performed could be observed, by students and colleagues who were seated around the central stage. The surgeons did not wear any specialized garments; surgeons simply wore ordinary aprons over their casual clothes. Surgeries were performed with bare hands in an unsterile environment. The importance of hygiene and asepsis was not strongly appreciated at that time. Health care workers did not wash their hands before examining or operating on patients. Incredibly, surgeons even failed to wash their hands after examining an infected corpse. Many doctors took pride in the accumulation of blood and pus on their medical garments.

Florence Nightingale, who came to be known as "The Lady of the Lamp," was a pioneer of modern nursing. Nightingale's most famous contribution came during the Crimean War. The wounded soldiers became her central focus after reports began to filter back to Britain about the horrific conditions. Nightingale and her compatriots believed that proper care should start with a thoroughly cleaned hospital and the equipment. She returned to Britain to begin to collect evidence for the Royal Commission on the Health of the Army. Nightingale believed that soldiers at the hospital died as a result of poor and unsanitary conditions. This experience would influence her later career; she advocated for the great importance of sanitary living conditions.

E-mail address: magerlm@wcmc.com

During the same time period, Joseph Lister (1827–1912), a professor at London's King College Hospital applied the knowledge of bacteria to develop a successful system of antiseptic surgery. Initially, Lister's achievements and findings were a matter of controversy because they were based on Pasteur's germ theory that was in dispute itself.

The recognition of the environment as a potential germ reservoir and as a source of contamination for the development of infection continues to gain in importance. During the 1990s, the US Department of Labor, Occupational Safety and Health Administration (OSHA) passed a regulation known as the Blood Borne Pathogen Standard. The standard required institutions to implement policies and procedures for the identification of potential exposure to bloodborne pathogens; and to implement a system designed to eliminate the potential for exposure of bloodborne pathogens to all health care workers. It required employers to ensure that worksites are maintained in clean and sanitary condition; the employer is also required to develop and implement an appropriate written schedule for cleaning. Furthermore, the employer must determine the method of decontamination based upon the location within the facility, type of surface to be cleaned, type of soil present, and tasks or procedures being performed in the area. In addition, all equipment, as well as environmental and working surfaces, must be cleaned and decontaminated after contact with blood or other potentially infectious materials. This would include decontamination with an appropriate disinfectant at the following times: after the completion of procedures; immediately–or as soon as feasible–after surfaces are overtly contaminated or after any spill

doi:10.1016/j.cpen.2008.01.007

of blood or other potentially infectious materials; and at the end of the work shift, if the surface may have become contaminated since the last cleaning [1].

The potential role of environmental reservoirs, such as surfaces and medical equipment, in the transmission of Vancomycin-resistant *Enteroccocci* (VRE) and other multidrug-resistant organisms (MDROs) has been the subject of several reports. MDROs are defined as microorganisms, usually bacteria, that are resistant to one or more classes of antimicrobial agents (ie, antibiotics). MDROs include: methicillin-resistant *Staphylococcus aureus* (MRSA); vancomycin-intermediate *Staphylococcus aureus* (VISA); vancomycin-resistant *Staphylococcus aureus* (VRSA); VRE; specific gram negative bacteria (GNB), including those producing extended spectrum beta-lactamases (ESBLs); and other organisms, such as *Escherichia coli* and *Klebiella pneumoniae,* that are resistant to multiple classes of antimicrobial agents. Additionally, MDROs include strains of *Acinetobacter baumannii* resistant to most antimicrobial agents; and *Sternotrophomonas maltophilia, Burkholderia cepacia,* and *Raistonia pickettii* that are intrinsically resistant to the broadest-spectrum antimicrobial agents [2].

Although environmental cultures are not routinely recommended, environmental cultures were used in several studies to document contamination. The studies led to interventions that included: the use of dedicated non-critical medical equipment; assignment of dedicated cleaning personnel to the affected patient care unit; and increased cleaning and disinfection of frequently touched surfaces [3]. In one study, an outbreak was noted in a burn intensive care unit (BICU) caused by VRE. After culturing such areas including overhead tables, bed rail, and monitors, approximately 13.5% of the cultures had grown VRE. Protocols were implemented including in-service training for hospital staff, including housekeeping personnel. Additional scheduled cleaning was implemented and a checklist was developed to ensure compliance. After all such changes were instituted, environmental cultures were negative and continued to be negative for over one year [4]. Another study addressed an outbreak of VRE in a neonatal intensive care unit (NICU). In this study, environmental samples were taken from area such as light switches, bassinet rails, and countertops. VRE was present in 16.7% of the samples. A more rigorous cleaning schedule was implemented and, after further environmental culturing, negative results were noted [5].

Different bacteria favor different conditions for growth and persistence. Dry conditions favor the persistence of gram positive cocci in dust and on surfaces, whereas soiled, moist environments encourage the growth and persistence of gram-negative bacilli. Fungi are also present in dust and they proliferate in moist, fibrous material [6].

A common reason given for finding environmental contamination with an MDRO is the lack of adherence to facility procedures for cleaning and disinfection. In an educational intervention that targeted a specific group of housekeeping personnel, there was a persistent decrease in the acquisition of VRE in a medical ICU [2]. Therefore, monitoring for adherence to recommended environmental cleaning practices is an important determinant for success in controlling the transmission of MDROs and other pathogens in the environment [2].

Surgical procedures interfere with normal skin protection and expose patients to microorganisms from either endogenous or exogenous sources. The prevailing standard of practice dictates that all patients be presumed to be infected with bloodborne and other pathogens. Consequently, any environmental cleaning in the surgical setting needs to minimize health care workers' and patients' exposure to potentially infectious microorganisms, including bloodborne pathogens.

The Association of Peri-operative Registered Nurses (AORN) developed "Recommended Practices for Environmental Cleaning in the Surgical Practice Setting," which was approved by AORN's board of directors and became effective January 1, 2003. The recommendations constitute the optimal level of practice; policies and procedures need to reflect the variations in the settings where they are used. This article concentrates on an acute care hospital setting [7].

All patients should expect that a safe and clean environment be provided in any health care institution. According to AORN's standards, the general environment of the OR should be cleaned on a routine schedule to ensure the reduction of the amount of dust, organic debris, and microbial load in this environment. ORs need to be cleaned routinely after each surgical procedure and they should be terminally cleaned at the end of the days' schedule. The most efficient process for meeting these standards is a team approach to cleaning. The team approach involves all members of the surgical team in the room turnover procedure; in assessing the degree of contamination; in deciding what needs to be cleaned; and acting appropriately. Such efficient teamwork in the room turnover process expedites the surgical schedule.

All horizontal surfaces in the OR (eg, furniture, surgical lights, and equipment) should be damp-dusted with an Environmental Protection Agency (EPA)-registered disinfectant before the start of the days schedule. The registered nurse in the OR acts as the advocate for the patient; the nurse has a responsibility to ensure that the environment is safe, free from dust and buildup on all horizontal surfaces, before creating the sterile field. All equipment from outside of the OR should be damp-dusted before entering the OR. This practice will reduce both the likelihood for the transmission of contaminants by the airborne route, and possible touch contamination from this equipment to the staff and or to the patient.

Items that may be contaminated should not leave the OR unless they have been subjected to some degree of decontamination. Partial cleaning, involving wiping down with an EPA-approved sanitizer, may only be feasible when the piece of equipment is necessary for urgent patient care procedures. All blood, tissue, and body-fluid specimens should be placed in leak-proof containers for the safe handling by health care workers. The outside surface of the specimen container received from a sterile field needs to be cleaned with an EPA-registered hospital disinfectant before the container leaves the environment of the OR. Such procedures reduce environmental contamination and result in an OR that is always relatively free of overt contamination.

Similarly, anesthesia equipment needs to be cleaned and processed according to AORN's recommended practices [7]. When cleaning, mechanical friction should be used because effective cleaning depends on the scrubbing actions and friction. The health of neonates is of particular concern because of their fragility and poorly developed immune systems. Disinfectant, antiseptics and other cleaning supplies may leave residue on the environmental surfaces which neonates may contact; adequate consideration and attention must be employed to avoid unnecessary exposure of neonates to these residues. The use of phenolics or any other chemical in bassinets or incubators is not recommended. If these types of solution are used, the bassinet or incubator must be thoroughly rinsed with water and dried before contact with the neonate.

At the end of the procedure, the team including the registered nurse, scrub personnel, surgeon, anesthesia personnel, and designated environmental services personnel should assess the immediate environment. Personnel should conduct spot cleaning before the room is prepared for the next case. Kick buckets should be emptied and sanitized; the OR table should be cleaned and sanitized; spot cleaning should be performed on the walls and on equipment showing evidence of contamination; and the floor around the OR table should be mopped clean. When routine cleaning is complete, the room is ready to be set up for the next case.

For each subsequent surgical case, a safe environment needs to be reestablished. As described previously, preparation of the OR should involve visual inspection and spot cleaning of visible contamination. There is no recommendation for high-level disinfection for environmental surfaces. Walls, doors, surgical lights, and ceilings should be spot cleaned in the event of being soiled with blood, tissue or body fluids. Visibly soiled areas on the floor should be cleaned using a new or freshly laundered mop head and an EPA-registered hospital-grade germicidal agent. The mop's head should be dipped into the solution only when the mop is clean, before the mopping activity, unless the germicidal agent is changed after use. Mops that are soiled or reused should not be re-dipped into the solution. If the floor is grossly contaminated and re-dipping is required, the solution will need to be changed to a fresh solution after use. The practice of floor cleaning removes the soil, organic debris, and dust. For end of procedure floor cleaning, a 3- to 4-foot perimeter around the surgical field should be cleaned only when the floor is visibly soiled. More extensive floor cleaning should occur only on areas where the floor is visibly soiled. The OR bed should be moved to check for such items as sponges and instruments that may have fallen into open spaces. Data does not support cleaning the entire floor after each case. However, during terminal cleaning the entire floor should be cleaned, including under the OR bed.

Because a clean surgical environment assists in the reduction of microorganisms, each surgical procedure room and scrub/utility area should be terminally cleaned at the end of the days' scheduled cases. An EPA-registered agent and mechanical friction need to be used to clean all areas that are listed below:

Surgical lights and external tracks
Fixed and ceiling-mounted equipment

All furniture and equipment, including wheels, casters, step stools, foot pedals, telephones, and light switches

Hallways and floors

Handles of cabinets and push-plates

Ventilation faceplates

Horizontal surfaces (ie, tops of counters, sterilizers, fixed shelving)

Substerile areas

Scrub and utility areas

Scrub sinks

During terminal cleaning, the OR floors should be wet-vacuumed with an EPA registered hospital disinfectant. This technique of mopping ensures that the cleaning solution is in contact with the floor for the proper amount of time (ie, according to the manufacturer's recommendation). Using a vacuum to remove the excess solution is not only effective, but also efficient. The practice assists in the decreasing the number of microorganisms in the surgical environment. The cleaning equipment must be taken apart and cleaned with EPA-approved hospital disinfectant. Cleaning equipment needs to be stored dry. These practices decrease the growth of bacteria during storage and reduces the possible contamination of the surgical suite.

There are no specific recommendations related to some areas and equipment in the surgical setting. However, during the terminal cleaning process, cleaning needs to be accomplished for the following:

Ducts and filters vents

Return ventilation and heating grilles

Recessed ceiling tracks

Closets

Cabinets

Shelves

Sterilizers

Warming cabinets

Refrigerators

Ice machines

Walls and ceilings.

A routine schedule of cleaning should be established for the unsterile areas, offices, lounges, lavatories, and locker rooms within the surgical suite.

The Centers for Disease Control and Prevention have identified environmental cleaning as one of the key factors in protecting patients from health care-associated infection. The cleaning of surfaces reduces the bioload in the environment.

The physical action of scrubbing with detergents and surfactants, followed by rinsing with water, removes a large number of microorganisms from surfaces. Most housekeeping surfaces require regular cleaning with a detergent or disinfectant and removal of soil and dust. Importantly, the employee should always refer to the manufacturers' instruction for appropriate use, dilution, and application methods of a cleaning product. In addition, alcohol should not be used to disinfect large environmental surfaces [3].

In each hospital, an interdisciplinary team should meet periodically to discuss the process of cleaning the operating rooms. New products and technologies for cleaning and sanitizing the environment continue to emerge; consequently, changes in the recommended process for cleaning the OR room may occur. Such changes need to be communicated to the entire surgical team. If changes in practice have occurred without the communicating them to clinical partners, then the efficiency of the cleaning process may be negatively impacted.

To facilitate the process of cleaning the OR, groups will need to meet periodically, at least annually, to identify if there are any changes in practices or if there are any changes with regulations or federal mandates. To ensure and facilitate the effectiveness of the cleaning procedures in the OR, team members should have the same understanding and expectations. The team members may include the following: OR staff; administration; Environmental Service Infection Control; anesthesia; and a representative from the surgical staff. Each member of the team should be able to articulate the definition of routine cleaning as compared with terminal cleaning.

Written policies and protocols lay the groundwork for all personnel to have the same understanding of the outcome expected. Errors should be kept at a minimum when there are written expectations. Monitoring for compliance with written policies can identify any lapses in practice or any changes in cleaning protocol.

The following is an example of what one may expect upon completion of the cleaning for between surgical cases:

1. The housekeeper will practice hand hygiene upon entering room.
2. The housekeeper will remove all trash and soiled linen, placing these items in a rolling cart to be transported to collection area outside of the OR. The rolling cart, with

collected trash/linen, is to be picked up from door of room by assigned housekeeping staff and transported to containers at the OR entrance.

3. Properly diluted quaternary ammonium solution and appropriate huck towel cleaning cloths are to be used for all disinfection procedures for routine, non-isolation cleaning between surgical cases. (Cleaning cloths are not to be double dipped into bucket of disinfectant; when cloth is used, it is to be thrown into linen hamper.) Cleaning solution must be changed between each room cleaning and clean huck towel cloths are to be used for each room. If double dipping occurs, cleaning solution must be changed; change cleaning solution as frequently as needed.

4. Disinfect all hand contact surfaces of overhead light to include handles, top and bottom of light, and swing arms.

5. Disinfect the surgical table thoroughly: wipe and disinfect all surfaces of mattress, the table surface under mattress, and all parts of the table using properly diluted quaternary ammonium solution. Remove and dispose of the table straps and replace them with new straps after each case.

6. Spot clean all vertical surfaces; check for visible soiling (ie, for blood or other body fluids or compounds) on all walls, ceilings, lights, and all other vertical and horizontal surfaces in the room.

7. Refill all appropriate dispensers in all areas including paper towel, antimicrobial soap, and hand sanitizer.

8. Re-line all trash and linen hampers.

9. Wash (ie, mop) floor with properly diluted quaternary ammonium solution.

10. Thoroughly check the room (eg, floors, equipment) to ensure all visible soiling is cleaned and room is ready for next case.

11. Practice hand hygiene upon exiting room.

An example of what one may expect for terminal cleaning:

1. Housekeeper will practice hand hygiene upon entering room.

2. The housekeeper will remove all trash and soiled linen and place them in a rolling cart to be transported to collection area outside of the OR. The rolling cart with collected trash and linen will be picked up from door of room by assigned housekeeping staff and transported to containers at entrance to the OR.

3. Properly diluted quaternary ammonium solution and appropriate huck towel cleaning cloths are to be used for all disinfection procedures for routine, non-isolation cleaning between cases. (Cleaning cloths are not to be double dipped into bucket of disinfectant; when cloth is used, it is to be thrown into linen hamper.) Cleaning solution must be changed between each room cleaning and clean huck towel cloths are to be used for each room; if double dipping occurs, cleaning solution must be changed.

4. Move all rolling stock to center of room.

5. Using a wall-washing tool, disinfect all high surfaces, including walls, overhead lights, medical gas hoses, and ventilation grills.

6. Wash (ie, mop) the circumference of room with properly diluted quaternary ammonium disinfectant solution.

7. For surface disinfection: wipe all horizontal and hand contact surfaces with properly diluted quaternary ammonium solution; clean OR door handles, tables, IV poles, buckets, blood pressure cuffs, monitor leads, bear hugger, tubes and the like; disinfect all rolling stock surfaces. All items should be cleaned using a "clean" to "dirty" technique, ie, cleanest, least soiled items shall be cleaned first, then proceed systematically to clean the most soiled items last.

8. Disinfect all rolling stock surfaces and equipment (including casters) and move equipment back to the perimeter of room. Disinfect all fixed equipment in the center of the room, including electrical cords and tubing.

9. Disinfect all interior scrub areas (ie, unsterile rooms) and sinks.

10. Disinfect the surgical table thoroughly, wiping and disinfecting all surfaces of the mattress, the table surface under the mattress, and all parts of the table using quaternary ammonium solution.

11. Refill all appropriate dispensers and replace the liners of waste receptacles with appropriate liners.

12. Practice hand hygiene upon exiting from the room.

Modifications to the recommended OR cleaning practice must be discussed. It is important to maintain the team concept by communicating with the population being served, recognizing the setting and the issues that may need to be addressed. The team must consider changes needed in the cleaning protocol in response to patients being on isolation more frequently with increased multidrug-resistant bacteria or newly emerging pathogens. This may occur if an endemic organism is identified that requires an alternative method of cleaning. In 2000, one urban university medical center identified an outbreak of a highly resistant ESBL positive, gram negative *Klebsiella pneumoniae*. It was reported that this organism was found to be tolerant to the quaternary ammonium compound and phenolics used in the hospital. However, it was discovered to be intolerant to a 1:5 bleach solution. A change in the cleaning solution was made to address this outbreak. Only an interdisciplinary team can address these types of issues be effectively [8].

In summary, general cleaning and terminal cleaning are important procedures in an OR. The role of the environment in the transmission of infection has not been directly identified, however, there have been health benefits achieved through environmental cleaning. The cleaning of surfaces decreases the bioload of surface contaminants and creates a health benefit by reducing the number of pathogens. The implementation of good procedures for cleaning and disinfecting frequently touched surfaces is well-documented. All personnel need to ensure, when caring for patients, that the environment is as safe as possible. To achieve the highest patient safety mandate, the cleanliness of the hospital environments is the best starting point.

References

[1] Department of Labor, OSHA. Occupational exposure to bloodborne pathogens: final rule. Federal Register, part II. 1991; CFR Part 1910.1030:64175. p. 64175–82.

[2] Siegel JD, Rhinehart E, Jackson M, et al. Management of multidrug-resistant organisms in healthcare settings 2007. Am J Infect Control 2007;35: S165–93.

[3] CDC. Guidelines for environmental infection control in health care facilities: recommendations of CDC and Healthcare Advisory Committee (HICPAC). MMWR 2003;52(RR10):1–42.

[4] Falk PS, Winnike J, Woodmansee C, et al. Outbreak of vancomycin-resistant Enterococci in a burn unit. Infect Control Hosp Epidemiol 2000; 21:575–82.

[5] Rupp ME, Marion N, Fey PD, et al. Outbreak of vancomycin-resistant *Enterococci faecium* in a neonatal intensive care unit. Infect Control Hosp Epidemiol 2001;22:301–3.

[6] Sehulster LM, Chinn RYW, Arduino MJ, et al. Guidelines for environmental infection control in health-care facilities, CDC, HICPAC, American Society for Healthcare Engineering/American Hospital Association, vol. 2004. Association of Operating Room Nurses. Recommended practices for sterilization in the perioperative practice settings. Standards, recommended practices and guidelines. Denver (CO): Association of Operating Room Nurses; 2006.

[7] Association of Operating Room Nurses. Recommended practices for sterilization in the perioperative practice settings. Standards, recommended practices and guidelines. Denver (CO): Association of Operating Room Nurses; 2006.

[8] Stokes C, Ingilma K, Magerl MA, et al. "Beyond Contact Precautions: Management of a Multi-Drug *Klebsiella pneumoniae* Outbreak in an Urban University Medical Center", to the APIC'01 28th Annual Educational Conference and International Meeting on June 12th, 2001 at Washington State Convention & Trade Center. Seattle, Washington.

ELSEVIER
SAUNDERS

Perioperative Nursing Clinics 3 (2008) 149–153

PERIOPERATIVE
NURSING
CLINICS

Multidrug-Resistant Pathogens: Implementing Contact Isolation in the Operating Room

Tania N. Williams, RN, MSN*, Janet P. Haas, RN, DNSc

Infection Prevention and Control Department, New York University Medical Center, New York, NY 10016, USA

Multidrug-resistant organisms (MDROs) are microorganisms that are resistant to commonly used antimicrobial agents [1]. Caring for patients who harbor MDROs while maintaining a safe environment for other patients and staff presents a challenge for the health care worker in the operating room (OR). Patients infected or colonized with MDROs require special preparations and precautions when scheduled for surgical procedures. Infection control measures must be tailored to the physical environment and to the characteristics of the patients served by the facility. Appropriate strategies must be fully implemented to reduce the risk of environmental contamination and subsequent transmission of MDROs to other patients [1].

Infection control principles

Understanding how infections are transmitted is essential to understanding the basic concepts of infection prevention and control. A "chain of infection" is necessary in order for infection to occur. The chain of infection includes a source; a mode or modes of transmission; a susceptible host; and a point of entry. In order for infection to be transmitted, each 'link' of the chain must be present [2].

Sources of infection may be infected or colonized patients, contaminated objects in the environment, or the hands of health care workers. Occasionally, faulty infrastructure systems are also implicated in the transmission of disease.

Examples of faulty infrastructure are contaminated water systems or air handling systems. Depending upon the organism, the environment plays a greater or lesser role in transmission. For example, vancomycin resistant enterococcus (VRE) may survive on surfaces for several days, so environmental cleaning plays a large role in containing this organism [3].

The classic routes of transmission for most disease are: airborne, droplet, or contact (direct and/or indirect) spread [2]. Vector-borne (via mosquitoes or ticks) transmission is not a concern in most health care facilities in developed countries. The most common route of transmission for MDROs is by contact with a contaminated person or object [2]. To prevent transmission, excellent hand hygiene practices, use of barriers for all patient care, and careful cleaning of equipment in the environment [1] must all be addressed.

Susceptible hosts are those at risk for acquiring infection. Although all people are susceptible to resistant bacteria, the amount of risk varies. Those at highest risk are the very young or very old, immunocompromised people, or people requiring extensive medical care [2]. In addition, living in communal situations, such as skilled nursing facilities [4] and prisons, or participation in contact sports [5] may also increase the risk of coming in contact with MDROs, and thereby increase the likelihood of becoming colonized or infected with them [2].

Points of entry include natural orifices (eg, mouth and nose), artificial orifices (eg, tracheotomy and colostomy), skin breaks, wounds, and mucous membranes. Invasive devices, such as intravenous catheters, indwelling urinary

---

* Corresponding author.

E-mail address: tania.williams@nyumc.org (T.N. Williams).

doi:10.1016/j.cpen.2008.02.003

catheters, and endotracheal tubes are also points of entry that breach the body's natural defenses. These devices provide microorganisms with opportunities to enter the body [2]. Large groups of bacteria may colonize the devices' artificial materials and create another risk of infection. In general, the use of invasive devices must be considered carefully and their use should be re-evaluated frequently. These devices should be removed as soon as possible to reduce the risk of infection.

MDROs such as VRE, methicillin-resistant *Staphlococcus aureus* (MRSA), and some resistant gram negative bacteria (GNB) require special infection control precautions called "Contact Precautions" [1]. Other organisms that are not drug-resistant, but that also require contact precautions include *Clostridium difficile*, a type of bacteria that causes intense colitis that may necessitate a colectomy. *C difficile* is easily spread in health care settings and therefore, it requires the same level of attention as MDROs [6]. Contact precautions require staff to take extra steps to ensure that these bacteria, which are easily transmitted by touch, are kept away from susceptible patients and staff. Contact precautions include: the use personal protective equipment (PPE), such as gowns and gloves; communication of patient's need for infection control precautions; careful cleaning of the environment; and strict adherence to hand hygiene protocols [1].

PPE is used when caring for any patient who needs contact precautions. The use of gloves and gowns for all patient contact is required; health care workers must anticipate when care of that patient will be needed. An example of anticipating patient needs in the OR is a circulator's recognition that help will be needed to transfer the patient from the stretcher to the OR bed. The circulator should be prepared with a gown and gloves to assist with this task. Masks and face shields are to be worn when splashing of blood or body fluid is likely [1]. In some institutions, masks are a regular part of contact precautions. In the OR, staff routinely wears masks, but eye protection is warranted if splashing is likely. PPE must be removed before leaving the patient area and before hand hygiene is performed.

Hand hygiene is the most significant act a health care worker can perform to reduce the risk of transmitting infection [7]. The Centers for Disease Control (CDC) recommends preferential use of alcohol-based hand sanitizing products for most situations [8]. The rationale is that alcohol-based sanitizers are easy to locate, since plumbing is not required, are less damaging to skin, and are more convenient for staff to use. Studies have correlated increased hand hygiene compliance with the availability of alcohol-based products and these have also been associated with decreases in MRSA [9]. Alcohol-based products do not remove soil from one's hands. Therefore, if hands are visibly soiled or feel sticky, hand washing with soap and water is the appropriate action. There is some controversy about the appropriateness of the use of alcohol-based products when caring for patients with *C difficile* because this bacteria forms spores that are resistant to alcohol. The latest CDC guidelines recommend using soap and water for these situations [6]. However, if soap and water are not easily available, alcohol-based products will kill some of the bacteria. One hospital reported no increase in *C difficile* rates when alcohol products were used with *C difficile*–infected patients [10].

Another way to reduce the risk of transmission of MDROs and *C difficile* is to avoid sharing equipment. If possible, the same stethoscope, blood pressure cuff, and other equipment used for contact precaution patients should be dedicated to that patient for his or her perioperative stay. When the patient leaves the holding area, this equipment may travel with the patient. If not, the equipment must be cleaned and disinfected before use on another patient. Similarly, environmental surfaces in the area must be cleaned and disinfected [1]. Most MDROs are killed by hospital grade disinfectants, if the disinfectants are applied and allowed to dry for the time recommended by the manufacturer. One exception is notable: *C difficile* spores are killed by bleach-containing products, but they are not killed by many other disinfectants [10]. Each facility should have protocols for cleaning equipment and the environment that takes these organisms into consideration.

Communication

In the OR, poor communication between health care workers may lead to adverse events that compromise patient safety [11]. Communication failure has been identified as the leading source of adverse events in surgery [12]. Communication failure may be a result of a problem originating from behavior and attitude, from systems, or from a combination of these. Safe, high quality performance is necessary to achieve optimal patient outcomes [13]. Breakdown in communication, beginning in the preoperative phase to the postoperative phase can significantly influence treatment and patient outcome.

Communication of a patient's need for contact precautions is essential to excellent and safe care. Patients known to harbor MDROs should be identified by the institution so that appropriate care can be given [1]. Many hospitals use their computer systems to flag these patients for current and future visits. For the surgical patient, the OR schedule may also be an appropriate place to note the patient's need for contact precautions. If the patient's condition and the OR schedule allow, the case may be planned for the end of the day or another time that is less busy [14]. This decreases the chance of inadvertently transferring resistant bacteria to other patients [14] and allows ample time for the cleaning staff to ensure that all equipment and surfaces in the OR are cleaned and disinfected after the case.

All levels of staff which provide care for the patient must be aware of the need for contact precautions. In addition to flagging the patient in the computer system and OR schedule, isolation precautions should be a part of the hand-off communication between nursing personnel. This verbal report helps ensure that the appropriate precautions will be taken. Preoperative briefings can inform all members of the team [12] of the patient's needs. Necessary non-sterile gowns and other PPE can be gathered before the patient arrives.

Anesthesia staff is integral to this process, as the patient's antibiotic prophylaxis may have to be altered based on having an MDRO [12]. If possible, include post anesthesia care unit (PACU) staff and cleaning personnel in any briefing. If this is not possible, include MDRO and contact precautions information in the hand-off communication from the OR to the PACU. Be sure to allow adequate time for the PACU to prepare for the contact precautions needed for the patient. This can be accomplished by either setting up the isolation room or by finding another appropriate location for the patient. Notify the cleaning personnel that the OR cleaning requires special attention to touched surfaces such as telephones; OR bed controls; anesthesia machine knobs; and the remainder of the OR furnishings and equipments.

Signage is another important way to communicate the patient's contact precautions need. Although transporter and receiving unit staff should know about the patient well in advance, signage on the patient's door and at the front of the patient's paper charts provide a fail-safe mechanism to convey the need for contact precautions. To ensure that teams know their roles, the institution may want to schedule a drill or audit one or more real cases. A checklist can be used to assess whether the patient's needs were documented in the computer, on the OR schedule, and given in the verbal report. Assess if there were disposable blood pressure cuffs and other equipment available, or if the team had the ability to quickly clean and disinfect equipment before the next patient's arrival. Assessing these items in an orderly manner can guide efforts for improvement.

Another method of improving communication among OR staff members is through the employment of Crew Resource Management (CRM) [12,13]. CRM is the use of all available resources such as information, equipment, and people to achieve safe and efficient care. This is a technique long-used in the aviation industry and it can be applied in the OR setting to improve communication. The framework for CRM program implementation includes: briefings; inquiry, advocacy, and assertion; self-critique; conflict resolution; and decision-making [13].

After adapting CRM, health care institutions have reported reductions in adverse outcomes, errors, and length of stay, along with improved nurse retention, and changed attitudes and behaviors toward teamwork [13]. Adoption of CRM in the OR suite can help to flatten hierarchies thereby eliminating perceived barriers to open discussion. It may also help to correct detrimental behavior patterns [13]. By focusing on improving systems rather than punitive actions for errors that occurs, CRM can create a healthy atmosphere in which staff feels a part of a team and members perform their duties safely, efficiently, and effectively [13].

Operative care

Caring for patients who harbor MDROs can be a challenge in the preoperative setting. Usually, patients wait for surgery in large, open holding areas, which is not ideal when the goal is to separate patients from one another. A strategy that can be used for inpatients is to call for them to the OR just before surgery, thus avoiding the holding area. For same day admission patients, there is no option to send for them immediately before their procedure. These patients can wait with others in general waiting areas unless they have respiratory symptoms or are otherwise unable to keep their secretions or excretions from contaminating the environment. Once the patient is changed and ready to go to the preoperative holding area, contact precautions should be used by health care workers. Workers should wear non-sterile gowns and gloves when contacting the patient or equipment that is used for that patient. Wearing PPE such as gowns and gloves when not in the sterile field is a change from normal OR practices that will primarily impact the circulator and anesthesia personnel. When assisting the patient onto or off of the OR table and when positioning the patient, staff should wear gowns and gloves. In some ORs, patient gowns used before the case are saved and used when the patient goes to the PACU. This practice should be altered for patients known to harbor MDROs; the potentially contaminated gown should be placed in the laundry bag rather than remaining in the OR throughout the case.

Anesthesia providers routinely wear PPE when inserting central lines, but wearing unsterile gowns for routine care of the patient is a change from their normal practice. While most of the patient is covered during surgery, it is important to remember that MRSA is most frequently found in patients' noses. It is certainly possible to contaminate hands and equipment when touching patients' faces.

During the actual surgical procedure, sterile gowns and gloves are used by the surgical team. Anesthesia providers should continue wearing gloves and gowns while providing care, and the circulator should be aware of any potentially contaminated items and wear appropriate PPE when contacting them. This should not be a big departure from standard practice. Traffic control in the OR is always recommended [15], but often not enforced. When the patient has an MDRO, not only does extra traffic increase the risk of a surgical site infection, but it also increases the chance that a staff member may carry an MDRO out of the room to other locations in the hospital. The surgeon and circulator should limit the number of extra personnel coming in and out of the OR during these cases. It is important to let the PACU team know that the patient needs contact precautions so that they can prepare a spot for the patient to be recovered. When the patient leaves the OR, the room should be cleaned and disinfected, including all surfaces and equipment that were touched by the patient or staff during the procedure.

Postoperative care in the PACU requires contact precautions, and patient placement again becomes an issue. Some facilities have an isolation room that can house patients who require contact precautions, but others have an open plan with no private area. In the latter case, the best strategy is to avoid putting the patient in the middle of the patient care area. Well-meaning staff may try to assist with patient care, and they may not realize that contact precautions are needed. Having the patient spatially separated is desirable to decrease the risk of sharing patient care equipment. If possible, dedicate staff members to the contact precautions patient's care. If this is not possible, the staff member caring for the patient who needs contact precautions must be keenly aware of the need to wear PPE for every patient encounter and to clean their hands before contacting any other patients.

In the future, more patients harboring MDROs may be identified as a result of screening cultures. MRSA, in particular, is an organism that is of interest preoperatively. Some surgeons screen for this bacteria and if an MRSA is found, the surgeons take steps to eradicate it before surgery. The surgeons may also change their prophylactic antibiotic agent. Some facilities have policies in place that require contact precautions for all patients who have ever been identified as having MRSA, however the risk of transmission from a patient in whom the bacteria has been eradicated before surgery should be quite low. Whether facilities require contact precautions for colonized or treated patients with no signs of active infection is the individual institution's decision.

Summary

Some patients who harbor MDROs need surgery as part of their care. This can be provided safely in the perioperative setting if staff members collaborate. Communication of the need for contact precautions is essential; real time information sets the stage for effective action [16]. Practice changes needed for contact precautions, such as use of gowns and gloves for all care, and dedicating and disinfecting equipment used in the holding area and PACU can be accommodated with appropriate advanced notice. It is difficult to measure the outcome of these efforts since patients do not stay in the perioperative setting long enough to develop signs and symptoms of infection [17]. However, auditing the process of care for these patients may help to identify areas for improvement.

Through proper coordination and collaboration of activities, risks can be minimized [18].

Dialog among OR personnel must be concise and relevant to promote clear and effective communication. There must be a shared mental model of how the patient encounter will proceed to promote the best possible patient care. Interventions to protect patients and the OR environment from contamination with MDRO and other microbes include the use of contact precautions along with traffic control, cleaning of equipment and the OR room after patient procedures, and dedication of equipment for use in the holding area and PACU. With good communication and attention to these details, patients who harbor MDROs can be cared for safely in the perioperative setting.

References

[1] Siegel JD, Rhinehart E, Jackson M. et al. Management of multidrug-resistant organisms in healthcare settings. The Hospital Infection Control Practices Advisory Committee and Centers for Disease Control, 2006. Available at: http://www.cdc.gov/ncidod/dhqp/pdf/ar/mdroGuideline2006.pdf.

[2] Dee M. Infection control. Nurs Stand 2000;14(28): 51–9.

[3] Bond WW, Favero MS, Petersen NJ, et al. Inactivation of hepatitis B virus by intermediate-to-high-level disinfectant chemicals. J Clin Microbiol 1983; 18(3):535–8.

[4] Raab U, Kahlau D, Wagenlehner F, et al. Prevalence of and risk factors for carriage of panton-valentine leukocidin-positive methicillin-resistant staphylococcus aureus among residents and staff of a German nursing home. Infect Control Hosp Epidemiol 2006;27:208–11.

[5] Centers for Disease Control and Prevention (CDC). Methicillin-resistant staphylococcus aureus infections among competitive sports participants–Colorado, Indiana, Pennsylvania, and Los Angeles county, 2000–2003. MMWR Morb Mortal Wkly Rep 2003;52(33):793–801.

[6] Siegel JD, Rhinehart E, Jackson M. et al. Guideline for isolation precautions: preventing transmission of infectious agents in healthcare settings. The Hospital Infection Control Practices Advisory Committee and Centers for Disease Control, 2007. Available at: http://www.cdc.gov/ncidod/dhqp/pdf/guidelines/Isolation2007.pdfwww.cdc.gov.

[7] Beyea SC. Keeping patients safe from infection. AORN J 2003;78(1):133–4.

[8] Boyce JM, Pittet D. Guideline for hand hygiene in health-care settings, vol. 15. The Hospital Infection Control Practices Advisory Committee and Centers for Disease Control, 2002. Available at: http://www.cdc.gov/mmwr/preview/mmwrhtml/rr5116a1.htm.

[9] Pittet D, Hugonnet S, Harbarth S, et al. Effectiveness of a hospital-wide programme to improve compliance with hand hygiene. Lancet 2000;356: 1307–12.

[10] Boyce JM, Ligi C, Kohan C, et al. Lack of association between the increased incidence of clostridium difficile-associated disease and the increasing use of alcohol-based hand rubs. Infect Control Hosp Epidemiol 2006;27:479–83.

[11] Horowitz IB, Horowitz SK, Brandt ML, et al. Assessment of communication skills of surgical residents using the social skills inventory. Am J Surg 2007;194:401–5.

[12] Awad SS, Fagan SP, Bellows C, et al. Bridging the communication gap in the operating room with medical team training. Am J Surg 2005;190(5): 1–7.

[13] Powell SM, Hill RK. My copilot is a nurse: using crew resource management in the or. AORN J 2006;83(1):178–202.

[14] Grota PG. Perioperative management of multidrug-resistant organisms in health care settings. AORN J 2007;86(3):361–8.

[15] Sehulster L, Chinn RY. Guidelines for environmental infection control in health-care facilities: recommendations and reports. The Hospital Infection Control Practices Advisory Committee and Centers for Disease Control, 2003. Available at: http://www.cdc.govmmwr/preview/mmwrhtml/rr5210a1.htm.

[16] Moss J, Xiao Y. Improving operating room coordination: communication pattern assessment. J Nurs Adm 2004;34(2):93–100.

[17] Tait AR, Tuttle DB. Preventing perioperative transmission of infection: a survey of anesthesiology practice. Anesth Analg 1995;80:764–9.

[18] Archer T, Macario A. The drive for operating room efficiency will increase quality of patient care. Curr Opin Anaesthesiol 2006;19:171–6.

ELSEVIER SAUNDERS

Perioperative Nursing Clinics 3 (2008) 155–161

PERIOPERATIVE NURSING CLINICS

Preventing Hepatitis B Transmission in the Perioperative Environment: Focus on Policies and Procedures

Lucille H. Herring, RN, MS, CIC

Weiler Division, Montefiore Medical Center, 825 Eastchester Road, Bronx, NY 10461, USA

Health care workers can become infected with the hepatitis B virus (HBV) through direct contact with blood or other potentially infectious materials (OPIM) during the performance of their duties. Vaccination is the best way to prevent transmission of hepatitis B in the perioperative setting. The next best thing is to have rational policies that are followed by all and are based on the Occupational Safety and Health Administration (OSHA) Bloodborne Exposure Standard. Other measures can include modifying work practices, reengineering needed sharps, and eliminating unsafe sharps in the health care environment. All levels of staff, including physicians, registered nurses, and surgical technicians, must be involved in the development of the policy, compliance with procedures and policies, and periodic review.

The virus

HBV is a small, double-shelled virus in the Hepadnaviridae virus family. The virus has a small circular DNA genome that is partially double-stranded. HBV contains numerous antigenic components, including hepatitis B surface antigen (HBsAg), hepatitis B core antigen, and hepatitis B antigen. The highest concentration of HBV is found in the blood and serum. Semen, vaginal fluids, and salvia can contain lesser concentrations of HBV. The only known hosts for HBV are humans [1].

Occurrence

HBV infection is a virulent infectious disease that causes inflammation of the liver, cirrhosis, and hepatocellular carcinomas. Worldwide, more than 350 million people are chronically infected with HBV. The incidence of acute hepatitis B has declined 75% from 8.5 per 100,000 people in 1990 to 2.1 per 100,000 people in 2004. The greatest decline (94%) has occurred in children and adolescents due to routine hepatitis B vaccination. HBV claimed an estimated 51,000 new cases in 2005. The highest rate of the disease occurs in 20- to 49-year-olds. The high risks groups for hepatitis B include persons who have multiple sex partners, men who have sex with men, intravenous drug users, sexual contacts, and close household contacts [2].

Clinical course

Clinical course of acute HBV is similar to that of other types of viral hepatitis. Approximately 50% of adults have asymptomatic acute infections. Others experience a nonspecific course of malaise, fever, aches, and pains (myalgia). There is a 3- to 10-day period before the onset of jaundice. There may be an onset of nausea, vomiting, anorexia, right upper quadrant abdominal pain, fever, headache, arthritis, skin rashes, and dark urine. The jaundice phase may last 1 to 3 weeks and exhibits jaundice, gray or light stools, and hepatic tenderness. The convalescence phase may last for weeks or months. Such symptoms as jaundice, fatigue, and malaise may persist for weeks or

E-mail address: lhhcon@aol.com

months. The incubation period is usually 45 to 180 days. All persons who are HBsAg positive are potentially infectious. Following acute HBV infection, the risk of developing chronic infection varies inversely with age [1].

Transmission

Health care workers can become infected with the HBV through direct contact with blood or OPIM during the performance of their duties. OPIM include but are not limited to semen, vaginal secretions, cerebral spinal fluid, synovial fluid, pleural fluid, peritoneal fluid, amniotic fluid, saliva, any body that is visibly contaminated with blood, and any unfixed human tissue or organ. Also, any blood tissue or organ from experimental animals infected with HBV, hepatitis C virus, or HIV is an OPIM. Transmission can occur through percutaneous or mucosal exposure. HBV can be transmitted from an infected mother to her baby, usually during the birthing process. The virus may be stable in dried blood on environmental surfaces for up to 7 days at 25° C. Hand contact with blood-contaminated surfaces may indirectly transfer the virus to skin or mucous membranes. In the perioperative area, spattering and some aerosolization of blood and bone fragments may occur during drilling and during the use of certain hand pieces and ultrasonic scalers [3].

It is estimated that 384,325 percutaneous injuries occur in health care workers annually [4]. Health care workers who perform invasive procedures are at high risk for injury. The operating room environment presents the greatest risks for these injuries. A survey of 17 medical centers involving 699 surgical residents about previous needlestick injuries, 99% of residents said they sustained a needlestick injury by their final (fifth) year of training. For 53% of the surgical residents, the injury involved a high-risk patient with a history of HIV, HBV, hepatitis C virus, or intravenous drug use. Fifty-one percent of the injuries were not reported to the employee health service. Lack of time was the most frequent (42%) reason given for not reporting such injuries [5]. These findings show that, to reduce needlesticks, there is a need for systems-based strategies, such as "sharpless" methods for handoff and passing instruments and needles, and innovative surgical techniques using nonsharp alternatives whenever possible. Improved reporting systems are needed. These could include needlestick hotlines, coverage

systems to facilitate prompt reporting, and peer education to create a culture that encourages speaking up.

Prevention policies

OSHA is an enforcement agency. In 1970, the OSHA Safety and Health Act of 1970, Provision Section 5(a) [1] was passed. This act's general duty clause states that an employer must maintain a workplace free from recognized hazards likely to cause death or serious physical harm to employees. OSHA can issue citations, track violations, and apply costly penalties under the general duty clause when hazards exist and are identified, even if no standards are issued. Table 1 presents a chronologic listing of standards, guidelines, recommendations, documents, and papers on prevention of transmission of bloodborne pathogens by different agencies and committees.

In 1991, OSHA issued its Bloodborne Exposure Standard, a standard related to occupational exposure to bloodborne pathogens [6]. This document is one of the most important policies ever written for preventing the transmission of blood and OPIM in the workplace. The OSHA Bloodborne Exposure Standard has led to changes in standards of practice and care in the health care industry and among state health departments; regulatory agencies, such as the Joint Commission; and professional organizations, such as the American Medical Association, the American Nurses Association, the Association of Perioperative Registered Nurses (AORN), the Association for Professionals in Infection Control and Epidemiology, and the Society for Healthcare Epidemiology of America.

The OSHA Bloodborne Exposure Standard states that every employer who has employees exposed to bloodborne pathogens must have a written exposure control plan designed to eliminate or minimize employee exposure.

According to the standard, the elements of the exposure control plan must contain at least the following elements:

- An exposure determination: Develop a written procedure to identify and classify all employee job classifications that may have occupational exposure to blood and OPIM.
- The schedule and determination of implementation: Methods of compliance include standard precautions to be used to prevent the bidirectional mode of transmission from

patient to health care worker. When work practice controls and engineering controls are in place and occupational exposure still exists, personal protective equipment will be used.

- Communications of hazards to employees: Warning (biohazard) tags, symbols, and signs must be properly affixed and displayed.
- Recordkeeping of the standard: Confidential medical records for each employee with occupational exposure must be maintained for the duration of the employee's employment plus 30 years. Employee training records shall be maintained for 3 years from the date on which the training occurred.
- HBV vaccination and postexposure evaluation and follow-up.

The perioperative area is a high-risk environment for exposure to hepatitis B and other bloodborne pathogens. OSHA requires every health care worker who may have any occupational exposure, defined to include any skin, eye, mucous membrane, or parenteral contact with potentially infectious materials on the job, be offered free of charge the hepatitis B vaccination. Each member of the staff in the perioperative area should be vaccinated against HBV at the start of his or her career. Susceptible unvaccinated perioperative staff members must be encouraged to receive the hepatitis B vaccination.

The vaccine is administered in a series of three shots. Vaccination against hepatitis B can be started at birth and provides long-term protection against infection in more than 90% of healthy

Table 1
Chronologic listing of standards, guidelines, recommendations, documents, and papers on prevention of transmission of bloodborne pathogens

Date	Document	Agency
1983	Guideline for Infection Control in Hospital Personnel	CDC
1991	U.S. Dept. of Labor, OSHA, Occupational Exposure to Bloodborne Pathogens: Final Rule, 29CRF Part 1910.1030, 1991	US Dept. of Labor, OSHA
1997	Immunization for Health Care Workers, MMWR (Vol. 46, No. RR-18)	CDC, ACIP, HICPAC
1998	Guideline for Infection Control in Health Care Personnel MMWR (Vol. 47, No. RR-19)	CDC
1999	Guideline for the Prevention of Surgical Site Infection	CDC, HICPAC
2001	Updated U.S. Public Health Service Guidelines For the Management of Occupational Exposures to HBV, HCV, and For Post Exposure Prophylaxis, MMWR, June 29, 2001/50 (RR-11)	CDC
2002	Guideline for Hand Hygiene in Health Care Settings: Recommendations for Health Care Infection Control Practices. Advisory Committee and the Task Force and the HICPAC/SHEA/APIC/IDSA Hand Hygiene Task Force	CDC, Hand Hygiene Task Force
2005	Updated U.S. Public Health Service Guidelines for the Management of Occupational Exposures to HIV and Recommendations for Post Exposure Prophylaxis MMWR, Sept. 30, 2005/54 (RR-09)	CDC
2005	Association of Perioperative Registered Nurses (AORN) AORN Guidance Statement: Sharps Injury Prevention In the Perioperative Setting. In: Standards, Recommended Practices and Guidelines, 2005: 199–204	AORN
2007	OSHA and NIOSH. Safety and Health Information Bulletin. Use of Blunt-Tip Suture Needles Decrease Percutaneous Injuries to Surgical Personnel. NIOSH Publication No. 2007–132	OSHA, NIOSH
2007	HICPAC 2007, Guidelines for Isolation Precautions: Preventing Transmission of Infectious Agents in Healthcare Settings, June, 2007	CDC

Abbreviations: ACIP, Advisory Committee on Immunization Practices; AORN, Association of Perioperative Registered Nurses; APIC, Association for Professionals in Infection Control and Epidemiology; CDC, Centers for Disease Control and Prevention; HCV, hepatitis C virus; HICPAC, Hospital Infection Control Practice Advisory Committee; NIOSH, National Institute for Occupational Safety and Health; SHEA, Society for Healthcare Epidemiology of America.

people. Any employee who refuses the vaccination must sign an informed refusal form.

There should be a postexposure evaluation and follow-up protocol. This protocol should include directives for the following actions:

1. Provide immediate care to the exposure site. Wash wounds with warm water. Flush mucous membranes with water.
2. Evaluate the exposure. Determine risk associated with the exposure (ie, blood and percutaneous injury).
3. Give postexposure prophylaxis for exposures posing risk of infection transmission. Give postexposure prophylaxis as soon as possible, preferably within 24 hours.
4. Perform follow-up testing and provide counseling. Advise exposed persons to seek medical evaluation for any acute illness occurring during follow-up.
5. Detail the procedures for the evaluation of circumstances surrounding exposure incidents [7].

In 2001, the Needlestick Safety and Prevention Act was passed. In response to this Act, OSHA revised the 1991 Bloodborne Standard. The revision states the need to select safer needle devices, to involve employee users in choosing such devices, and for employers to maintain a log of injuries from contaminated sharps [8].

Personnel in the perioperative area are at high risk for exposure to bloodborne pathogens. Operating room personnel are at high risk for transmission of bloodborne pathogens when passing sharps instruments. In 2005, the AORN published in the AORN Journal the AORN guidance statement Sharps Injury Prevention in the Perioperative Setting [9]. The perioperative-specific risk-reduction strategies called for in this statement are listed in Box 1.

Suture needles

In 2005, the American College of Surgeons (ACS) issued a statement supporting universal adoption of blunt-tip suture needles for suturing fascia. The ACS stated that all published studies to date have demonstrated that the use of blunt suture needles can substantially reduce or eliminate needlestick injuries from surgical needles [10].

In 2007, OSHA, the Department of Labor and National Institute for Occupational Safety and Health, the Centers for Disease Control and Prevention, and the Department of Health and Human Services developed a Safety and Health Information Bulletin titled, "Use of Blunt-Tip Suture Needles to Decrease Percutaneous Injuries to Surgical Personnel." This document describes the hazard of sharp-tip suture needles as a source of percutaneous injuries to surgical personnel. Sharp-tip suture needles are the leading source of percutaneous injuries to surgical personnel, causing 51% to 77% of these incidents [11]. Sharp-tip suture needles not only injure surgical staff, but also present a risk to patients from potential exposure to blood from an injured staffmember. Blunt-tip suture needles are effective in decreasing percutaneous injuries in surgical personnel, especially when used to suture muscle and fascias. The use of blunt-tip suture needles complies with OSHA'S requirement to use safer medical devices where clinically appropriate.

Masks

Surgical masks are medical devices regulated by the Food and Drug Administration. OSHA, under 29 CFR 1910.1030 Bloodborne Pathogens, Final Rule, requires the use of face shields, masks, and eye protection if there is a possibility of occupational exposure to blood and OPIM. AORN states that surgical masks should be worn at all times in the operating room and in environments where open sterile supplies or scrubbed personnel may be located. Masks are worn at all times in the restricted area of the operating room where sterile supplies are opened, in clean cores, and at scrub sinks. Masks with face shields or masks and protective eyewear are required whenever splash, spray, or aerosol of blood or OPIM may be generated. Masks in combination with eye protection devices, such as glasses with solid eye shields or goggles, or chin-length face shields, should be worn whenever splashes, spray, spatter, or droplets of blood or OPIM may be generated and eye, nose, or mouth contamination can be reasonably anticipated. Personal eyeglasses are not considered eye protection devices unless they have side shields. Masks should be secured to prevent venting [12].

Barrier gowns

The aseptic barrier materials for surgical gowns are classified as Class II Medical Devices by the Food and Drug Administration. The American Society for Testing Materials (ASTM) uses two tests—one for liquid penetration and one for viral penetration—for determining the

Box 1. Perioperative-specific risk-reduction strategies from the AORN Sharps Injury Prevention in the Perioperative Setting guidance statement

Work practice controls

Adopt and incorporate safe habits into daily work activities when preparing and using sharp devices.

Focus attention on the intent of the action when working with sharp items, and minimize rushing and distractions while applying safety techniques during critical moments.

Work practice controls during preparation for operative or other invasive procedures

Inspect the surgical field for adequate lighting and space to perform the procedure.

Organize the work area so that the sharps are always pointed away from staff members.

Use standardized sterile field set-ups.

Include identification of the neutral zone in the perioperative briefing, during communication handoff, and during shift change. The neutral zone is a safe zone for passing sharps, including scalpels and needles. Policies may be established requiring the use of a kidney basin in which the sharps is placed, the use of a designated area on the sterile field, or the use of the word "sharps" when passing these instruments.

Engineering controls during the operative or other invasive procedure

Contain used sharps on the sterile field in a designated, disposable, puncture-resistant needle container, and replace it as necessary.

Check to be sure the disposable, puncture-resistant needle container is securely closed before handling it off the field.

Encourage the use of blunt suture needles.

Personal protective clothing during the operative or other invasive procedure

Masks

Barrier gowns

Gloves

Work practice controls during the operative or other invasive procedure

Use neutral or hand-free technique for passing sharp items whenever possible or practical, instead of passing hand-to-hand.

Give verbal notification when passing a sharp device.

Keep visual contact with the procedure site and the sharp device.

Take steps to control the location of the sharp device.

Load suture needles using the suture packet to assist in mounting the suture needle holder, and use the appropriate instrument to adjust and unload the needle.

Remove the needle from the suture before tying or use control-release suture that allows the needle to be removed with a straight pull on the needle holder.

Be aware of other staff members in the area when handling a sharp device.

Keep track of and account for all sharp items throughout the procedure.

Activate the safety feature of a safety engineer device immediately after use according to the manufacturer's instructions.

Keep hands away from the surgical site when sharp items are in use (eg, during suturing, cutting).

Provide a barrier between the hands and the needle after use.

Use gloves and an instrument to pick up sharp items (eg, suture needles, hypodermic needles, scalpel blades) that have fallen on the floor.

Work practice controls during postprocedure cleanup

Inspect the surgical setup used during the procedure for sharps.

Avoid bringing hands close to the opening of a sharps container.

Do not place hands or fingers into a container to dispose of a device.

Keep hands behind the sharp tip when disposing.

Transport reusable sharps in a closed, secure container to the designated cleanup area.

Engineering controls during postprocedure cleanup

Inspect the sharps container for overfilling before discarding disposable sharps in it.

Make sure the sharps container is large enough to accommodate the entire device.

From Association of periOperative Registered Nurses. AORN guidance statement: sharps injury prevention in the perioperative setting. AORN J 2005;81:665–6; with permission.

effectiveness of protective clothing [13]. The materials are rated on a pass/fail basis. Manufacturers of materials can market their products as impervious/liquid-proof if the products pass both tests. The ASTM's mission is to reduce the risk of occupational exposure to bloodborne pathogens. The tests still do not identify the material's limitations. There is still a need for an inexpensive test to assess a product's protective capabilities [14].

Gloves

Surgical gloves are also regulated as medical devices and are regulated by the Food and Drug Administration. The ASTM sets the gloves standard. The acceptable quality level pinhole rate is 1.5 for surgical gloves. This means the defect number for 1000 gloves cannot exceed 15 or 1.5% of the total glove batch [15]. Remember to monitor gloves for punctures.

Surgical gloves must comply with the OSHA Bloodborne Pathogen Standard and provide an adequate barrier against HBV and HIV. In choosing a surgical glove, the following must be taking into account: glove length, thickness, tear resistance, elasticity, allergen content, and powder content. Surgical gloves are made from natural rubber latex, neoprene, or polyisoprene. The new glove technology has added protective coatings to the inside of the glove. These coatings help to keep the skin moist and intact.

Two layers of surgical gloves (double gloving) can decrease the number of breaks to the innermost glove that might allow cross-infection between the surgical team and patient. Double gloving does not affect surgical performance. Double gloving is becoming more common, especially for surgery where sharp surfaces are found, such as orthopedic or dental surgery. Research has shown that glove liners and extra thick gloves further reduce breaks to the inner glove [15].

Summary

In the preoperative environment, the modification of engineering and work practice controls to eliminate or decrease exposure to bloodborne pathogens is the foundation of today's perioperative nursing. The OSHA Bloodborne Exposure Standard has stimulated manufacturers of health care products to develop technology to catch up to the needs of the health care industry. Zero tolerance of exposure to bloodborne pathogens can be achieved through following the OSHA

Bloodborne Exposure Standard, modifying work practices, reengineering needed sharps, and eliminating unsafe sharps in the health care environment. All levels of staff, including physicians, registered nurses, and surgical technicians, must be involved in the development of the policy, compliance with procedures and policies, and periodic review. Vaccination is the best way to prevent transmission of hepatitis B in the perioperative setting. The next best thing is to have rational policies that are followed by all and are based on OSHA Bloodborne Exposure Standard.

References

[1] Heyman DL, David. Control communicable diseases manual. 18th edition. American Public Health Association; 2004. p. 143–4.

[2] Centers for Disease Control and Prevention. Surveillance for acute viral hepatitis—United States. Morbidity and Mortality Weekly Report 2007; 56(SS03):10–1.

[3] Taylor DL, David. Bloodborne pathogen exposure in the OR—What research has taught us and where we need to go. AORN J 2006;83(4):834–43.

[4] Panlilo AL, Orelien JG, Srivastava PU, et al. Estimates of the annual number of percutaneous injuries among hospital-based healthcare workers in the United States, 1987–1998. Infect Control Hosp Epidemiol 2004;25:556–62.

[5] Makary MA, Martin, Al-Attar, et al. Needlestick Injuries among surgeons in training. N Engl J Med 356:2693–8.

[6] U.S. Department of Labor. Occupational Safety and Health Administration, Bloodborne Pathogens Standard (29CFR 1910.1030). Fed Regist 1991;56: 64003–182.

[7] Centers for Disease Control and Prevention. A comprehensive immunization strategy to eliminate transmission of hepatitis B virus in the United States: recommendations of the advisory committee on immunization practices (ACIP) part II: immunization of adults. Morbidity and Mortality Weekly Report 2006;55(RR16):2–3.

[8] Centers for Disease Control and Prevention. Recommendations for preventing transmission of human immunodeficiency virus and hepatitis B virus during exposure-prone invasive procedures. MMWR Morb Mortal Wkly Rep 1991;40:1–9.

[9] Association of Perioperative Registered Nurses (AORN). AORN guidance statement: sharps injury prevention in the perioperative setting. In: 2005 standards, recommended practice and guidelines; 2005. p. 199–204.

[10] American College of Surgeons (ACS). Statement on blunt suture needles. Bull Am Coll Surg 90(11):24.

[11] Tanner J, Parkinson H. Double gloving to reduce surgical cross-infection. Cochrane

Database Syst Rev 2006;(3):CD003087. doi: 10. 1002/14651856.

[12] Davis Philip, Spady Donald, Forgie Sarah. A survey of Alberta physicians' use of and attitudes toward face masks and face shields in the operating room setting. Am J Infect Control 35(7):445–59.

[13] Belkin Nathan. The new standard for barrier surgical gowns and drapes: What it means to the infection control practitioner. AORN J 2006;.

[14] Belkin Nathan. AORN, OR gowns—even a "pass" can fail. AORN J 1999.

[15] Thomas Jane, Jensen Lori. Surgical glove performance: choosing an optimal surgical glove and understanding the performance criteria, managing infection control. 2007;52–8.

ELSEVIER
SAUNDERS

Perioperative Nursing Clinics 3 (2008) 163–169

PERIOPERATIVE
NURSING
CLINICS

Emergency Surgery on a Patient Who Has Infectious Tuberculosis

George Allen, RN, PhD, CNOR, CIC[a],*,
Kevin Caldwell, RN, BSN, CNOR[b]

[a]*Downstate Medical Center, 450 Clarkson Avenue, Box 1187, Brooklyn, NY 11203-2056, USA*
[b]*Consortium of Workers Education, 275 7th Avenue, 6th Floor, New York, NY 1001, USA*

The perioperative milieu, particularly the operating room setting, is generally viewed as an environment in which therapeutic interventions are performed on patients to return them to wellness. This environment also can subject patients and personnel to negative outcomes, however, such as surgical site infections [1,2], transmission of blood-borne pathogens [3,4], transmission of multi-drug–resistant pathogens, including methicillin-resistant *Staphylococcus aureus* [5,6] and the transmission of numerous other communicable diseases that are spread by contact or through the respiratory system [7], including tuberculosis (TB) [8]. Generally, preventing the transmission of blood-borne pathogens, including hepatitis B and other pathogens such as methicillin-resistant *Staphylococcus aureus* that are spread through the contact route, is fairly easily accomplished in the operating room because it is facilitated by the universal application of aseptic technique and compliance with the Occupational Safety and Health Administration blood-borne exposure standard, which requires the use of barriers when contact with blood and other potentially infectious materials is anticipated [9]. Surgical team members use scrupulous attention to maintaining a sterile field, displaying a surgical conscience and adhering to rigorous standards of asepsis during the perioperative period. When the infection is spread through the airborne route, however, as with TB, then planning,

prompt notification, and modification of some standard procedures are required. Perioperative managers must be prepared to provide appropriate settings to safely perform emergency surgical procedures on patients who may have a communicable disease or condition that is transmitted through the airborne route.

Tuberculosis

TB is an often severe and communicable bacterial (causative agent, *Mycobacterium tuberculosis* [MTB]) disease spread by the airborne route. TB typically affects the lungs but also may affect any other organ of the body. It is usually treated with a regimen of drugs taken for 6 months to 2 years, depending on the type of infection. For someone to develop active TB disease, the following two events must take place:

The bacteria must enter the body, thereby causing an MTB infection. This usually happens when a person breathes in MTB-contaminated air and the inhaled TB bacteria make their way to the lungs.
The immune system cannot stop the TB bacteria from growing and spreading after the initial infection.

Worldwide, more than 8 million people develop active TB annually, and approximately 2 million die from the disease each year. The World Health Organization estimates that more than 14 million people are living with TB. In 2005, out of an estimated 8.8 million new TB cases worldwide, 629,000 cases involved HIV-positive persons. An

---

* Corresponding author.
E-mail address: george.allen@downstate.edu
(G. Allen).

1556-7931/08/$ - see front matter © 2008 Elsevier Inc. All rights reserved.
doi:10.1016/j.cpen.2008.02.005

estimated 1.6 million people died of TB in 2005, 12% of whom were co-infected with HIV. TB and HIV/AIDS form a lethal combination, each speeding the other's progress. Because HIV weakens the immune system, someone who is HIV/TB co-infected is many times more likely to become sick with TB than someone infected with TB who is HIV negative [10].

It is estimated that more than one third of the world's population has the TB bacterium in their bodies, which means that they have MTB infection. Fortunately, only a fraction of people infected with MTB develops active TB disease. Individuals who do not get sick are known to have noncontagious latent TB, so called because the bacteria are inactive. TB bacteria can remain in this dormant state for months, years, and even decades without increasing in number and without making the person sick. Most people with latent MTB infection test positive on the tuberculin skin test or their chest radiograph shows signs of latent TB.

The TB skin test, also known as the Mantoux test, is performed by injecting 0.1 mL of tuberculin, purified protein derivative, intradermally in the upper aspect of the arm. The skin reaction is read 48 to 72 hours later. A positive or negative test result is reported depending on the size in millimeters of the induration seen. A positive reaction is generally defined as an induration of more than 10 mm. For people who are HIV positive, a reaction of 5 mm or more is considered positive. A newer test using a blood sample recently became available. Positive findings indicate that the TB germ is in the person's body, but most infected people do not develop active TB disease, may never get sick, may never show any symptoms, and may never spread the bacteria to others. One in ten people infected with TB bacteria does develop active TB disease, however.

People with weakened immune systems (eg, individuals with HIV disease, those receiving chemotherapy, or children younger than 5 years of age) are at a greater risk for developing TB disease. When they breathe in TB bacteria, the bacteria settle in the lungs and start growing because the individual's immune system cannot fight the bacteria. In these people, TB disease may develop within days or weeks after the infection. In other people, however, TB disease may develop months or years after the initial infection, at a time when the immune system becomes weak for other reasons and is no longer able to fight the bacteria. When a person gets active TB, it means that the TB bacteria are multiplying and attacking the lungs or other parts of the body, such as the lymph nodes, bones, kidney, brain, spine, and even the skin. From the lungs, the TB bacteria move through the blood to different parts of the body.

Symptoms of active disease include persistent cough, chest pain, loss of weight and appetite, fever, chills, and night sweats and symptoms from the specific organ or system that is affected (eg, coughing up blood or sputum in TB of the lungs or bone pain if the bacteria have invaded the bones). TB disease usually can be cured with prompt and appropriate treatment, but it remains a major cause of death and disability in the world, particularly among persons infected with HIV. Appendix 1 provides some additional general information on TB.

Preventing tuberculosis transmission

Airborne precautions are designed to reduce the transmission of diseases spread by the airborne route. Airborne transmission occurs by the dissemination of either airborne droplet nuclei (evaporated droplets) or small particles in the respirable size range (1–5 μm) that contain the infectious agents and remain airborne and viable for several days. Infectious agents spread by this route include *Aspergillus spp*, rubeola virus, the varicella-zoster virus, and *M tuberculosis*. Patients diagnosed with or suspected of having these pathogens must be cared for in airborne infectious isolation rooms, a single room that has a monitored negative airflow pressure and is often referred to as a negative-pressure isolation room. Personnel who enter the room must don a personal health care respirator (eg, N 95) mask (Fig. 1). When a patient is suspected of having or diagnosed with infectious TB, the current recommendations require that the patient be cared for in an airborne infection isolation room with negative pressure in relation to the corridor, and the door should remain closed unless someone is entering or leaving.

Operating room pressure differential

Current recommendations require that operating rooms be maintained under positive pressure in relation to the corridors [11]. In a positive-pressure room, when the door is opened, the air from inside the room rushes out into the corridor. The result is that potentially contaminated air from

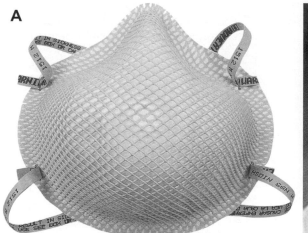

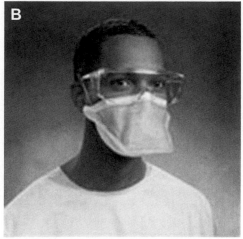

Fig. 1. N95 respirators suitable for use in the operating room. (*A*) 1500 N95 series respirator. (*Courtesy of* Moldex-Metric, Inc., Culver City, CA; with permission.) (*B*) Another N95 respirator. (*Courtesy of* Kimberly-Clark Worldwide, Inc., Dallas, TX. Copyright © Kimberly-Clark Worldwide, Inc. Used with permission.)

the corridor does not enter the room while the patient is known to be exceptionally at risk for the transmission of infections (eg, an incision is open). If the room is under negative pressure in relation to the corridor, the reverse occurs. Air from the corridor flows into the room when the door is opened. Consequently, a patient with active infectious TB who has surgery in a positive-pressure operating room can be an infectious source of the TB bacteria for individuals outside of the room whenever the door is opened unless additional special precautions are taken. Box 1 outlines recommendations for preventing the transmission of TB in the surgical suite when a negative-pressure operating room is not available.

Case scenario

A 25-year-old man who had recently returned to the United States after living and studying in Asia for 4 years was admitted to the hospital because of night sweats, fever, and weight loss of 18 lb (8 kg) within 3 months. The patient also reported a productive cough with sputum production. On admission to the hospital, the patient's temperature was 37.4°C, heart rate was 120 beats/min, and blood pressure was 126/80 mm Hg. The respiratory rate was normal, but breath sounds were diminished in the lower parts of the left lung, and a few crackles were heard bilaterally. Pulmonary TB was suspected. The patient

was placed into airborne precautions, a purified protein derivative was placed, chest radiographs were obtained, and sputum was collected for acid fast bacilli three times. (The specimens were collected at least 8 hours apart.) Chest radiograph revealed bilateral infiltrates, and the acid fast bacilli smear results were positive.

The patient was placed on anti-TB medication. After 24 hours in the hospital, he developed periumbilical pain and vomiting, his pulse was 160 beats/min, his temperature was 38.6°C, and blood test revealed an elevated white blood cell count of 12.6. Physical examination of the abdomen revealed appreciable direct tenderness over the right iliac fossa, particularly over McBurney's point, voluntary guarding, and rebound tenderness. Based on the history of vomiting and abdominal pain and the signs of direct lower quadrant tenderness and rebound tenderness with an elevated white blood cell count, the patient was diagnosed with acute appendicitis and booked for emergency surgery. Prompt appendectomy has long been the standard of care for acute appendicitis because of the risk of progression to advanced pathology and postoperative complications. This standard was recently validated during a retrospective review of 1081 patients who underwent an appendectomy for acute appendicitis. The results revealed that in adult patients with acute appendicitis, the risk of developing advanced pathology and postoperative complications increases with time. The authors concluded that delaying appendectomy is unsafe [12].

Box 1. Recommendations for preventing the transmission of tuberculosis in surgical suites

Administrative controls
Schedule a patient with suspected or confirmed TB disease for surgery when a minimum number of health care workers and other patients is present and as the last surgical case of the day to maximize the time available for removal of airborne contamination.
For postoperative recovery, place the patient in a room that meets the requirement for an airborne infection isolation room.

Environmental controls
If a surgical suite has an operating room with an anteroom, that room should be used for TB cases.
If surgery is needed, use a room or suite of rooms that meets requirements for an airborne infection isolation room.
If an airborne infection isolation room or comparable room is not available for surgery or after operative recovery, air cleaning technologies (eg, high-efficiency particulate air filtration and ultraviolet germicidal irradiation) can be used to the number of equivalent air changes per hour.
Bacterial filters should be used routinely in breathing circuits of patients suspected of or confirmed as having TB disease and should filter particles 0.3 μm in size in an unloaded and loaded situation with filter efficiency of > 95%.

Respiratory protection controls
For health care workers present during surgery of a patient with suspected or confirmed infectious TB disease, at least N95 disposable respirators, non-valve, should be worn.
Standard surgical or procedure masks for health care workers might not have fitting or filtering capacity for adequate protection.
If a patient has signs or symptoms of infectious TB disease (ie, positive acid fast bacilli sputum smears result),

consider having the patient wear a surgical mask, if possible, before and after the procedure.
Valve or positive-pressure respirators should not be used because they do not protect the sterile surgical field.

———

From the Centers for Disease Control (CDC) and Prevention. Guidelines for preventing the transmission of *Mycobacterium tuberculosis* in health care settings. MMWR 2005;54(RR-17:1–121).

Preparing for surgery

The patient was placed on the emergency list as an addition to the day's operating room schedule. In booking the patient, the physician notified the operating room manager that the patient had a diagnosis of pulmonary TB and required emergency surgery for acute appendicitis. The operating room manager noted that the last scheduled case of the day was expected to be completed at 4 PM and that operating room #6—one of two operating rooms with an anteroom—would be available. She confirmed that all the staff members on duty, including personnel who would be assigned to the case, had been fit tested and certified to wear the N95 non-valve respirator. She also ensured that the respirators were readily available. The anesthesia care providers were again notified of the patient's diagnosis and were reminded that bacterial filters should be used on the expiratory limb of the ventilator or anesthesia machine. (To prevent contamination of the anesthesia machine, a high-efficiency particulate air filter should be placed between the Y-connector and the mask, laryngeal mask airway, or endotracheal tube.)

Coordinating the care with the medical and nursing staff on the unit, the patient wore a surgical-type mask, bypassed the holding area, and was transferred directly to the operating room where the surgical procedure was to be performed. All the supplies and equipment needed for the procedure were already in the room, which reduced the potential for the door to be opened during the procedure. All personnel in the room, including the surgeon, anesthesia care providers, nurses, and surgical technicians, were wearing the N95 valve-less health care respirator mask.

Table 1
Air changes per hour and time required for removal
efficiencies of 99% and 99.9% of airborne contaminants

ACH	99%	99.9%
	Minutes required for removal efficiency[a]	
2	138	207
4	69	104
6	46	69
12	23	35
15	18	28
20	14	21
50	6	8
400	<1	1

Abbreviation: ACH, air changes per hour.
[a] Time in minutes to reduce the airborne concentration by 99% or 99.9%.
Data from CDC. Guidelines for preventing the transmission of *Mycobacterium tuberculosis* in health-care settings, 2005. MMWR Recomm Rep 2005;54(RR–17).

After the appendix was removed and the incision closed, the patient was extubated and recovered while still on the operating room table. He was subsequently transferred while wearing a surgical mask directly to his negative-pressure isolation room, bypassing the postanesthesia care unit. The operating room was left vacant so that it would be cleared of MTB (see the chart in Table 1) before it was cleaned and prepared for the next surgical procedure. In general, most operating rooms operate at a minimum of 15 air changes per hour. Consequently, the room should have been left vacant for approximately 30 minutes before anyone who was not wearing the N95 respirator mask entered.

Summary

All health care institutions should have a TB control plan that includes protocols for maintaining a high index of suspicion for patients being admitted with infectious TB, procedures for the early recognition of such patients, procedures for adequate room assignments, including airborne infection isolation room, procedures for screening personnel for infectious TB, and procedures for the annual fit testing and certification of personnel who may come in contact with or have to care for patients suspected of having or diagnosed with infectious TB to wear the N95 health care respirator. The N95 respirator is designated as the applicable respiratory protective personal protective equipment that must be worn by personnel

when infectious TB is suspected. Perioperative managers must ensure that they are always prepared to perform surgery on a patient with a communicable disease spread through the airborne route. Recognizing that recommendation when the disease is TB includes

Scheduling the case at the end of the day's schedule whenever possible so that individuals such as personnel and staff are potentially exposed as little as possible

Using an operating room with an anteroom, if available

Having staff wear non-valve N95 respirators

Keeping the doors to the operating room closed during the procedure, except for entry and exit of personnel

Leaving the room vacant before reusing, depending on number of air changes per hour

Appendix 1

Fact sheet

Tuberculosis: general information last updated: July 2007

What is tuberculosis?

TB is a disease caused by germs that are spread from person to person through the air. TB usually affects the lungs but can also affect other parts of the body, such as the brain, kidneys, or spine. A person with TB can die if he or she does not get treatment.

What are the symptoms of tuberculosis?

The general symptoms of TB disease include feelings of sickness or weakness, weight loss, fever, and night sweats. The symptoms of TB disease of the lungs also include coughing, chest pain, and coughing up blood. Symptoms of TB disease in other parts of the body depend on the area affected.

How is tuberculosis spread?

TB germs are put into the air when a person with TB disease of the lungs or throat coughs, sneezes, speaks, or sings. These germs can stay in the air for several hours, depending on the environment. Persons who breathe in the air containing these TB germs can become infected, which is called latent TB infection.

What is the difference between latent tuberculosis infection and tuberculosis disease?

People with latent TB infection have TB germs in their bodies but are not sick because the germs are not active. These people do not have symptoms of TB disease and cannot spread the germs to others. They may develop TB disease in the future, however. They are often prescribed treatment to prevent them from developing TB disease.

People with TB disease are sick from TB germs that are active, meaning that they are multiplying and destroying tissue in the body. They usually have symptoms of TB disease. People with TB disease of the lungs or throat are capable of spreading germs to others. They are prescribed drugs that can treat TB disease.

What should I do if I have spent time with someone who has latent tuberculosis infection?

A person with latent TB infection cannot spread germs to other people. You do not need to be tested if you have spent time with someone with latent TB infection. If you have spent time with someone with TB disease or someone with symptoms of TB, however, you should be tested.

What should I do if I have been exposed to someone who has tuberculosis disease?

People with TB disease are most likely to spread the germs to people they spend time with every day, such as family members or coworkers. If you have been around someone who has TB disease, you should go to your doctor or local health department for tests.

How do you get tested for tuberculosis?

Two tests can be used to help detect TB infection. The Mantoux tuberculin skin test is performed by injecting a small amount of fluid (called tuberculin) into the skin in the lower part of the arm. A person given the tuberculin skin test must return within 48 to 72 hours to have a trained health care worker look for a reaction on the arm. A second test is the QuantiFERON-TB Gold test. The QuantiFERON-TB Gold test is a blood test that measures how the patient's immune system reacts to the germs that cause TB.

What does a positive tuberculin skin test or QuantiFERON-TB Gold test mean?

A positive tuberculin skin test or QuantiFERON-TB Gold test only tells that a person has been infected with TB germs. It does not tell whether the person has progressed to TB disease. Other tests, such as a chest radiograph and a sample of sputum, are needed to see whether the person has TB disease.

What is Bacille Calmette-Guérin?

Bacille Calmette-Guérin (BCG) is a vaccine for TB disease. BCG is used in many countries but is not generally recommended in the United States. BCG vaccination does not completely prevent people from getting TB. It may also cause a false-positive tuberculin skin test result. Persons who have been vaccinated with BCG can be given a tuberculin skin test or QuantiFERON-TB Gold test, however.

Why is latent tuberculosis infection treated?

If you have latent TB infection but not TB disease, your doctor may want you to take a drug to kill the TB germs and prevent you from developing TB disease. The decision about taking treatment for latent infection is based on your chances of developing TB disease. Some people are more likely than others to develop TB disease once they have TB infection, including people with HIV infection, people who were recently exposed to someone with TB disease, and people with certain medical conditions.

How is tuberculosis disease treated?

TB disease can be treated by taking several drugs for 6 to 12 months. It is important that people who have TB disease finish the medicine and take the drugs exactly as prescribed. If they stop taking the drugs too soon, they can become sick again; if they do not take the drugs correctly, the germs that are still alive may become resistant to those drugs. TB that is resistant to drugs is harder and more expensive to treat. In some situations, staff of the local health department meet regularly with patients who have TB to watch them take their medications. This is called directly observed therapy, which helps patients complete treatment in the least amount of time.

This material was last reviewed on March 18, 2007.

From Centers for Disease Control and Prevention. Division of tuberculosis elimination. National Center for HIV/AIDS, Viral Hepatitis, STD, and TB Prevention. 2007. Available at: http://www.cdc.gov/tb/pubs/tbfactsheets/tb.htm.

References

[1] Lee JT. A new surgical site infection (SSI) prevention guideline. Surg Infect (Larchmt) 2000;1(2):127–31.

[2] Babkin Y, Raveh D, Lifschitz M, et al. Incidence and risk factors for surgical infections after total knee replacement No 9. Scand J Infect Dis 2000;39:890–5.

[3] Heptonstall J, The Incident Investigations Teams, et al. Transmission of hepatitis B from 4 infected surgeons without hepatic B e antigen No 3. N Engl J Med 1997;336:178–87.

[4] Carman WF, Cameron SO. What should be done about hepatitis B infected healthcare workers? J Med Microbiol 2003;52:371–2.

[5] Nelson J. Microbial flora on operating room telephones No 3. AORN J 2006;83:607–23.

[6] Hartnick CJ, Shotts S, Willging JP, et al. Methicillin resistant *Staphylococcus aureus* otorrhea after tympanostomy tube placement. Arch Otolaryngol Head Neck Surg 2000;126:1440–3.

[7] Chow T. Ventilation performance in operating theaters against infections: review of research activities and practical guidance No 2. Journal of Hospital Infections 1980;56:85–92.

[8] Centers for Disease Control and Prevention. Guidelines for preventing the transmission of Mycobacterium tuberculosis in health-care settings. MMWR 2005;54(RR-17):1–121.

[9] Occupational Safety and Health Administration. Occupational exposure to blood borne pathogens final rule. Federal Register 1991;29 CFR part 1910, 1030 56(253):64175–64182.

[10] WHO. Global tuberculosis control: surveillance, planning, financing. Geneva (Switzerland): WHO; 2007.

[11] Mangram AJ. Hospital Infection Control Advisory Committee (HICPAC) and Centers for Disease Control and Prevention (CDC). Guidelines for prevention of surgical site infection. Infect Control Hosp Epidemiol 1999;24(4):247–78.

[12] Ditillo MF, Dziura JD, Rabinovici R. Is it safe to delay appendectomy in adults with acute appendicitis? Ann Surg 2006;244(5):656–60.

ELSEVIER
SAUNDERS

Perioperative Nursing Clinics 3 (2008) 171–174

PERIOPERATIVE
NURSING
CLINICS

Index

Note: Page numbers of article titles are in **bold face** type.

1556-7931/08/$ - see front matter © 2008 Elsevier Inc. All rights reserved.
doi:10.1016/S1556-7931(08)00036-3

periopnursing.theclinics.com